For my LCIE family; staff, clients, colleagues, and pals.

Laura Thomas PhD, PgDip, RNutr is a Registered Nutritionist
and Director of the London Centre for Intuitive Eating (LCIE).
Laura established LCIE in 2017 to help support clients who have a
difficult relationship with food and their body. She has a passion
for delivering inclusive, trauma-informed, and person-centred
care for all bodies. She draws upon different therapeutic and
counselling skills to support her clients in their recovery from
disordered eating, chronic dieting, and body dissatisfaction.
In 2019 Laura published her first book *Just Eat It: How Intuitive
Eating Can Help You Get Your Shit Together Around Food* with
Bluebird, Pan Macmillan. She is also host of the podcast Don't
Salt My Game. Laura has a PhD in Nutritional Sciences and a
postgraduate diploma in Eating Disorders and Clinical Nutrition.

LAURA THOMAS PhD

How to
JUST
EAT IT

A step-by-step guide to escaping diets and finding
FOOD FREEDOM

bluebird
books for life

First published 2021 by Bluebird
an imprint of Pan Macmillan
Pan Macmillan, The Smithson, 6 Briset Street, London, EC1M 5NR
Associated companies throughout the world
www.panmacmillan.com

ISBN 978-1-5290-4369-3

9 8 7 6 5 4 3 2 1

A CIP catalogue record for this book is available from
the British Library.

Printed and Bound in Italy

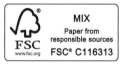

Visit **www.panmacmillan.com** to read more about all our books
and to buy them. You will also find features, author interviews and
news of any author events, and you can sign up for e-newsletters
so that you're always first to hear about our new releases.

CONTENTS

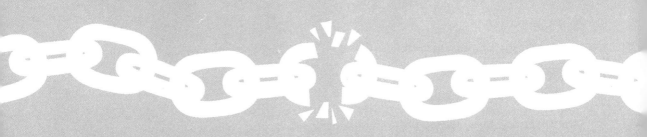

INTRODUCTION

In 2019, I published my first book, *Just Eat It: How Intuitive Eating Can Help You Get Your Shit Together Around Food*. Dolly Alderton called it 'truly life-changing' – so, ya know, no biggie! The book was a culmination of everything I'd learned in my formal nutrition training, plus a whole bunch of stuff I had learned working with actual humans. In my practice, the London Centre for Intuitive Eating (LCIE), myself and my team of nutrition counsellors help people navigate complicated or troubled relationships with food and their body. We use a lot of tools from the Intuitive Eating framework, but also pull in helpful nuggets from other frameworks and modalities to best support our clients.

In the years since I wrote the book, my work and practice have grown; I've learned new tools and new skills and gained more experience helping people apply this stuff in their lives. I wanted to incorporate many of the new tools I've learned into this workbook to give you a comprehensive companion for helping to heal your relationship with food and your body. I've also had loads of requests from readers of *Just Eat It* wanting more practical tools and exercises they could work through to help deepen their intuitive eating practice, sparking the idea for a workbook. Intuitive eating makes a lot of logical sense, but actually applying it is a whole other ball game.

HOW DID WE GET HERE?

Soon after starting my freelance nutrition practice, I noticed something I hadn't seen before (or maybe hadn't wanted to see!). People were coming to me for help with nutrition but were trying to refine, optimize, or otherwise 'perfect' their eating. They bought into the idea of good foods and bad foods and felt enormous stress and guilt if they 'slipped up' and ate anything from the latter category. Clients would berate themselves over the smallest dietary transgressions and double down on *what else* they could cut out of their diets; sugar, dairy, gluten, nightshades, meat, eggs, soy, peanuts – there was basically nothing left to eat! To be clear, there was no underlying allergy or intolerance for these folks, just deeply ingrained messages about 'right' and 'wrong' foods that were inherited from wellness gurus and influencers at a time when 'clean eating' was the diet du jour.

Clean eating, and the wellness culture it inspired, is of course just a spin-off from its insidious older sibling, diet culture. A belief system of patriarchal values that encourages people (particularly women, but increasingly folks of all genders) to believe that their bodies are not good enough as they are. It's a set of cultural programming that teaches us we need to pursue weight loss, diets, and 'the perfect body', with as much commitment and dedication as our families, careers, and relationships. When we stop to take a beat, we start to notice that diet culture messaging is everywhere, preying on our insecurities and vulnerabilities with made-up problems like cellulite and stretch marks, and then conveniently selling us back the solution at a premium. We don't stop to notice the small print: diets don't work. Even if we've learned this a million times over from trying every diet going, diet culture convinces us it's our fault. That we are the failures, even though diet companies bank on our repeat business. We just need more willpower, more self-control, to go to more groups, get the apps and wearable fitness trackers, buy the 'recipe' books (which let's face it is being generous), sign up to the online courses, and of course get a coach and trainer. Maybe then we'll lose that 'baby weight'?

Diet culture robs us of our time, energy, money, headspace, and other valuable resources. It keeps us locked into body hatred and the pursuit of weight loss at the expense of nurturing other passions. It glamorizes disordered eating, normalizing the restriction of whole food groups and vilifying innocuous ingredients. In *The Beauty Myth*, Naomi Wolf famously wrote, 'Dieting is the most potent political sedative in women's history; a quietly mad population is a tractable one.' In other words, we are so distracted by solving the so-called problems of our bodies that we can't engage in wider activism and social justice issues outside of ourselves. Diet culture destroys our relationship with food and our bodies; we overthink every food choice, we have to 'earn' or 'make up' for everything that passes our lips, we treat food and exercise like a maths equation rather than things that enhance how we engage in the rest of our lives. Now, at LCIE, I work with people to help them get unstuck from the clutches of diet culture and body shame, and help them build a more positive relationship with food and their bodies using the tools and principles of intuitive eating and similar frameworks, many of which I'm going to share with you here. But first up . . .

WHAT IS INTUITIVE EATING?

Imagine if you could eat (and actually enjoy!) the foods that you like, without shame, guilt, or frustration. Imagine if the voice in your mind that bargained and negotiated with you about 'making up' for eating a cookie by going on an extra-long run or eating less the next day just *shut the hell up*. Imagine if you could move your body for pleasure, fun, and play rather than punishment. Imagine you could feel complete and total liberation from food rules, body hate, and diet prison. Imagine you felt peace and freedom around food and your body. Imagine if you had the headspace to think about and do the things that were really meaningful and fulfilling to you.

I know it sounds almost too good to be true, but this is what Intuitive Eating has to offer. Most of us are born with strong connections to our physical hunger and satiety cues and use those cues to help guide our eating as babies. But that attunement to our bodies becomes deteriorated through living in diet culture which instils us with food rules, guilt, and shame that serve to undermine our intuition. The result? We end up in patterns of disordered eating: never-ending diets, being 'good' one minute and 'blowing it' the next, severely limiting the types of food we eat in order to eat 'clean', counting our macros and more; disordered eating takes many guises, but the bottom line is that the worse our relationship with food, and the more disordered our eating, the farther we are from

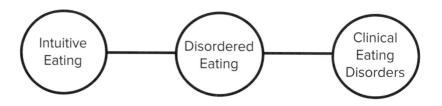

HOW TO JUST EAT IT

eating intuitively. You can imagine it on a spectrum; on one end we have clinically diagnosed eating disorders that require professional treatment. Then we have disordered eating, which can and does lead to eating disorders, and which deserves help and support in its own right. Then at the far end of the spectrum, we have intuitive eating; eating free from rigid rules, restrictions and guilt. Instead, intuitive eating invites us to make peace with forbidden foods and give ourselves unconditional permission to eat the foods we enjoy and that satisfy us. It encourages us to tap into our innate biological signals for hunger and fullness and to find pleasure and a sense of well-being from food. It brings forbidden and so-called 'bad' foods down off a pedestal so we can approach them all neutrally, without being emotionally or morally charged.

Even if we are not on a formal diet, we might be on a pseudo-diet, a lifestyle plan that is really just a diet in disguise; or perhaps all of our food choices are guided by external rules that we have accumulated over time ('no carbs after 6' or 'fats are "bad"'). For shorthand, I'm lumping these all together as 'diets' in the book.

Intuitive eating might feel out of reach after a lifetime of food rules and giving over our self-worth to the scales, but only because diet culture has indoctrinated us into thinking there is only one option available to us: micromanage our food, our bodies, and our weight, or risk being ostracized. We are promised we'll be better, happier humans once we reach an elusive body ideal, and when that promise is never delivered on, we blame ourselves. We become stuck in the diet cycle, going round and round, further eroding our self-esteem with each turn. Intuitive eating is the off-ramp to a healthier relationship with food and our bodies.

Intuitive eating has had a lot of buzz over the past few years, but it's not actually a new concept! The intuitive eating framework was developed back in the mid-1990s by two registered dietitians – Evelyn Tribole and Elyse Resch. These two pioneers noticed that sending people off with a calorie-controlled meal plan worked for a bit . . . but then further down the line, their clients were coming back full of self-blame and shame about 'not having enough discipline' or 'not having enough willpower'. Being the compassionate practitioners they are, Tribole and Resch realized that there had to be a better way to support their clients. So they did what any savvy nutrition professional would do and turned to scientific literature for answers. They quickly realized that there was a whole line of scientific enquiry supporting their clinical observations: people tend to regain weight after a diet. The science was pretty clear on this. Taking what they could glean from the literature, they decided to create a new framework for helping people let go of dieting, make peace with food, and find body respect. Thus, intuitive eating was born. At its creation, intuitive eating was an evidence-informed programme, meaning that although it took its cues from the scientific evidence that was available at the time, there were no studies directly measuring its impact. The cool thing is, some twenty-odd years later, intuitive eating is an active area of research, with scientists researching the benefits across wide groups of people (I'll fill you in on the benefits of IE in a bit!).

The thing about Evelyn and Elyse is that as the science develops, and their understanding deepens, they aren't afraid to update their model and incorporate new tools, techniques, and ideas. As it stands, the intuitive eating model is a set of ten overarching principles. The word *principle* is intentional and deliberate, because the idea is to help guide and support you to find what is best for you, rather than dictate and command what you 'should' do. Intuitive eating is designed to be flexible and approachable, not rigid and prescriptive like dieting. Fundamentally, it's about unlearning external diet and food rules, and learning to eat from a place of self-care.

This is how intuitive eating's architects, Evelyn and Elyse, define it:

Intuitive Eating is a self-care eating framework, which integrates instinct, emotion, and rational thought, and was created by two dietitians – Evelyn Tribole and Elyse Resch – in 1995. IE is a weight-inclusive, evidence-based model with a validated assessment scale and over 120 studies to date.[1]

These are the 10 principles of Intuitive Eating:[2]

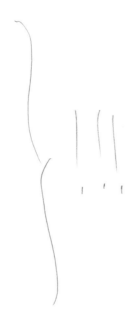

1   Reject the Diet Mentality

2   Honour Your Hunger

3   Make Peace with Food

4   Challenge the Food Police

5   Discover the Satisfaction Factor

6   Feel your Fullness

7   Cope with Your Emotions with Kindness

8   Respect Your Body

9   Movement – Feel the Difference

10 Honour Your Health – Gentle Nutrition

WHAT ARE THE BENEFITS?

Like I said, intuitive eating is a really active area of research (I'm even involved in a research project in the NHS!). But it's important to remember that it's still a relatively new line of enquiry, so we don't have everything figured out just yet. That said, the initial studies are promising. Intuitive eating seems to support health both physically and emotionally/psychologically. Here's the breakdown:

Physical

* Can support blood glucose control, helping prevent and manage diabetes (including gestational diabetes).[3-8]

* Can support heart health; early studies suggest that intuitive eating can help lower blood pressure, low-density lipoprotein ('bad') cholesterol and triglycerides, and can help increase high-density lipoprotein ('good') cholesterol.[9-11]

* Can help people eat a more varied and nutritious diet (this is especially important to remember considering people sometimes equate intuitive eating with being the 'screw it, eat whatever you want' diet).[12]

Emotional/psychological

* Intuitive eating is associated with less disordered eating practices like dieting, fasting, and skipping meals. It's also associated with reduced symptoms of bulimia nervosa, anorexia nervosa, and binge-eating disorder.[13-16]

* Intuitive eaters seem to have higher body appreciation and body satisfaction and less body surveillance.[13, 17]

* Intuitive eaters are more likely to have better mood overall.[16]

HOW IS THIS BOOK DIFFERENT?

I've had the enormous privilege to train with and learn from Evelyn and Elyse (and they've both been on my podcast!); I owe them both an enormous debt for their work and for shaping my career – without their work I'm pretty sure I'd still be stuck in a calorie-counting, 'perfect-eating', weight-centric nutrition practice (even the thought makes me feel weird!). But ultimately, I'm not them.

This book is my spin on intuitive eating; it reflects the way I practice, and is shaped by my clients, the people who have generously shared their stories and experiences with me. I'm also not an intuitive eating purist; while intuitive eating is my bread and butter and forms the backbone of this book, I'm also bringing in tools, techniques, and ideas from other modalities. In particular I draw a lot on Acceptance and Commitment Therapy or ACT, a set of tools that *— look into* beautifully complements the intuitive eating framework. You'll see a lot of ACT-informed work in Chapter 1 – Laying the Foundation: Your Intuitive Eating Toolkit. This section is designed to give you a set of fundamental skills and tools that you can lean on when the going gets tough. You can think of this book as my take on intuitive eating, with some other supportive strategies, concepts, and tools brought in to help you. And seeing as this is a workbook, I'm also focusing a lot more on the *practice* rather than the theory and encouraging you to do your own research using this book to guide you.

In my practice, I take the OG ten principles of intuitive eating and give them the remix treatment. They are my interpretation of the principles, if you like. I've added bits and removed others, trying to keep true to the spirit and intention of intuitive eating.

I've laid out the concepts in the same order that I work through with my clients. I'd encourage you to work through them in this order initially, and then go back and review sections that you're feeling a bit stuck with or need a refresher on.

This book is broken down into twelve chapters:

There's also an appendix at the back with additional tools and templates we'll use throughout the book, plus, I'm sharing some of my favourite further resources so you can continue deepening your intuitive eating practice. Each chapter is accompanied by a corresponding podcast where you'll find more conversations, tools and support to help guide you. Search Don't Salt My Game in your podcast app and look out for the episodes starting *How to Just Eat It*.

WHO IS THIS BOOK FOR?

People who want to develop a healthier relationship with food and their body: If you've struggled with disordered eating, hating your body, or been on some sort of diet for as long as you can remember, then I hope this book will help you find peace with food and let go of dieting for good.

People in eating disorder recovery: If you have an active eating disorder, then the tools in this book can help guide you back to a place where you're eating instinctively, rather than on the terms of an eating disorder. But not all of these concepts are appropriate at every stage in recovery and you may have to go through a period of more structured eating until you're physically and psychologically well enough to lean into intuitive eating. I've indicated which concepts, principles, and tools are appropriate throughout ED recovery (regardless of which ED you're in recovery from), and which might need to be saved until later. Ask your treatment team to help you navigate this, and make it clear that intuitive eating is the goal of your recovery. There's no harm in learning all there is about intuitive eating to help support your recovery (if that's a goal of recovery for you), even if you can't fully apply it yet.

Clinicians and counsellors: If you're a nutritionist, dietitian, therapist, or anyone else supporting people to heal their relationship with food and their body, then I hope you can use this book as a guide with your clients. However, please remember that intuitive eating and working with disordered eating/eating disorders is a specialist area and requires appropriate professional training and ongoing clinical supervision. See https://londoncentreforintuitiveeating.co.uk/for-healthcare-professionals for more on how we can support you in this work.

HOW TO USE THIS BOOK

Before we jump in, let's slow things down and figure out how to get the most from this book.

Take your time: Seriously. Cool your jets. When people are struggling to 'get' intuitive eating, it's usually because they're trying to rush to the finish line. So trust me when I say, there's no finish line, there's no certificate, there's no medal. Slow your roll. And try and enjoy the process; the more we can sink down into it, instead of forcing it, the easier we will find it. 'Getting' intuitive eating is actually pretty anticlimactic: it sort of just becomes normal and boring.

Do the work: This is a workbook. Workbook is code for 'I'm-going-to-make-you-work-for-it-book'. This isn't me trying to be a hardass, or passing the buck. It's because intuitive eating is not a passive process. The clients who have the most success are the ones who do their own research and learning between sessions; doing the activities is obviously going to be part of that, but an equally important part is noticing, reflecting, and making sense of the information in the context of your own life. It's easy to understand intuitive eating rationally and intellectually; it's what we were born knowing. But unlearning body shame and the rules of diet culture takes effort. People often assume that intuitive eating means 'eat when you're hungry and stop when you're full', but if you're only focused on these elements, you're missing out on the full expression of intuitive eating, meaning its flexibility, nuance, and shades of grey. Some of the work isn't easy, or all that fun, but it's important to stick with it, even if it's uncomfortable and challenging. Therefore, I invite you to actually do the reflections, and answer the journaling questions – don't just skim over them.

Look out for symbols

I've indicated different types of exercises with different symbols:

 means a guided meditation script – you can either record it yourself on your phone, or ask a friend or family member.

 indicates an opportunity for reflection and contemplation; I'm inviting you to write down responses to questions or prompts – you'll probably want to use a notebook or journal to have extra space to write in.

 is a reminder to check out the accompanying podcast with myself and special guests.

 indicates that there's further action required to complete the activity.

> **A word on trauma:** I'm no therapist, but I can appreciate that many people who struggle in their relationship with food and their body may have experienced some form of trauma in their lives. I've done my best to be sensitive to this, but I can't know all the different ways this might manifest for you, what you might find triggering or what it might bring up for you. I do, however, trust you to look after yourself, and if you feel overwhelmed by any of the practices or activities, please seek out professional support. If this isn't available to you, then talk with a trusted friend or loved one, or reach out to an online or IRL community to hear about other people's experiences.

Stick a pin in the pursuit of weight loss: Intuitive eating is not a diet, but we can sometimes approach it with the same mentality as we did a diet. This can do us a disservice: if our primary objective is weight loss, which is an external, appearance-related goal, it can undermine our ability to tap into and trust our bodies' cues. How can we respond to hunger, for example, if we are simultaneously trying to eat less? It can inadvertently draw out the intuitive eating process and keep us feeling a bit stuck. Intuitive eating doesn't judge or blame anyone for wanting to lose weight, but it does invite us to challenge our beliefs around the relationship between health, beauty ideals, fitness, and weight. It's OK if you feel the pull of weight loss (it's hard not to in this culture), but try and dig a little deeper and be curious about what's behind that. The activities in Chapter 2 will help break down diet mentality.

Don't sweat nutrition: For many of us, the only time we've paid attention to nutrition is when we are embarking on a new diet or lifestyle programme. If we're not careful, we can weaponize nutrition and turn it into another thing to beat ourselves up about if we don't do it perfectly. But here's the thing: there is no such thing as a perfect food or a perfect diet. Gentle nutrition is intentionally left until the end of the intuitive eating process; this is because we need to break down all-or-nothing, black-and-white thinking before approaching nutrition concepts. Making peace with food and giving ourselves unconditional permission doesn't just mean with cakes and pastries, but also with foods that we might have usually associated with dieting (and consequently maybe overdone it on). It can take time to get there, so remember that what we eat in the short term isn't going to have an impact on our long-term health; there's a lot of work ahead in challenging our (often mis-)conceptions about nutrition, and putting nutrition into perspective. Try not to sweat nutrition.

WHAT TO EXPECT FROM THE PROCESS

People often come to intuitive eating with the expectation that once they stop dieting, they are then eating intuitively.

Not. So. Fast.

Intuitive eating is a process, with ups and downs. You don't just say one sentence in French and then declare yourself fluent. It's the same deal with intuitive eating: it's a skill (or set of skills, really) that you learn to integrate over time. My brilliant colleague Marci Evans uses the analogy of a string of fairy lights to describe this process. Most people expect there to be a light bulb moment where suddenly everything is super clear, but it's more like a string of fairy lights that slowly turn on, one by one. And if you're looking ahead at all the tiny lights that are yet to go on, it's easy to lose sight of all the tiny lights that have already come on behind you. This speaks to the importance of reflecting on your experiences, and noticing the little shifts as well as the big wins.

It's also realistic to keep some perspective over how long the process might take, and to give yourself the time and space to let intuitive eating fully integrate into your life. I cannot tell you the number of times I've had a frustrated client sat in front of me questioning why it isn't working. Not only will I encourage them to look back at all the fairy lights that have already switched on for them, but I'll ask them how long they have spent dieting. The answer varies depending on the age of the client, but for some people it's upwards of twenty, thirty or forty years. I'll follow up by asking, 'How long have you been practising intuitive eating?' It might be a matter of weeks or months, but even if it's been a couple of years, it's usually only a drop in the bucket compared to the dieting days. I don't say this to scare you or freak you out. It's a reminder to slow down and let it sink in. Just because it may take some time to totally kick those lingering diet-y thoughts doesn't mean you won't notice some big changes in the short and medium term.

How long have you spent dieting, worrying about what, when, and how much you eat, or trying to manipulate your body through diet and exercise? How does this compare to how long you've been practising intuitive eating?

For many of you coming to this book, this may be the first time you've experimented with intuitive eating. Remember that it takes time to develop new skills and that the time you've spent with intuitive eating is likely a fraction of the time you've been following strict food rules and trying to lose weight. It's helpful to keep this in mind if you ever hear your critical voice try and tell you that you're not doing it right, or you should just quit now. Give yourself permission to *be a beginner*.

THE STAGES OF INTUITIVE EATING

Intuitive eating might look, feel, and work differently for different people; this means that the process of getting there will likely look different too, but I wanted to give you a sense of what you might expect, based on how I've see it play out for my clients. Please note that this is not a linear process and you might go back and forth between the various different stages or be at more than one simultaneously. Just know that it's all OK, however this process works out for you.

The mind-blown phase

This is likely where a lot of you are now, or at least soon will be once we get into it. This is the moment where you've been rudely and abruptly woken up to the damage that dieting has caused you personally, and the injustice and suffering it has contributed to vulnerable communities and marginalized groups, and you feel an urgency to let *everyone* know. This is the 'Intuitive Eating Evangelist' stage where you feel deep aggression and rage at your best friend for mentioning the D word to you and want to stage protests outside the *Women's Health* magazine offices. I get it. And I think the passion, energy, and intensity are great, but it's important to conserve your energy. There will be time for activism and angst. Let yourself find your feet first. Giving yourself a solid foundation will bring you longevity with this work.

The honeymoon phase

This is the term coined by the wonderful Christy Harrison to describe the freedom and highs of being able to eat *whatever you want*. For some people this feels like a fun and liberating place to hang out. Others can feel they're out of control. Either way, it won't last forever, so try and enjoy it. I'll also do my best to step you through it so it feels manageable rather than overwhelming.

The second-guessing everything stage

This is where you might start questioning whether you'll ever be able to 'get' intuitive eating. You get stuck in your head and question every choice you make about food and exercise. You might notice shifts in your behaviour but still have a lot of shit talk going on from your inner critic – this is totally normal. This voice can take some time to pipe down but eventually it will become a distant whisper.

The meltdown

Everyone has a wobble with intuitive eating. Some people might throw their arms up and walk away. Some people might even flirt with one last diet. This is a normal part of the process. Breathe, remind yourself why you came to intuitive eating in the first place. Find community (online or IRL) to share your concerns with, or get support from a Certified Intuitive Eating Counsellor if it would help. Also it's useful to do some reflection here, too – go back and reread the 'Your Relationship with Food' section in Chapter 2.

The starting to get it phase

You're beginning to notice those little shifts in how you feel about food and your body. Maybe you're noticing the extra headspace for engaging in bigger things. Maybe you're feeling a bit more confident wearing that figure-hugging dress, or notice yourself feeling calmer and more relaxed around food. Maybe your self-esteem and mental health are better. Because these shifts might feel more subtle than numbers changing on a scale, it's essential to slow down and tune into them.

The 'what's the big deal?' phase

Intuitive eating has fully integrated into your life: it's not something you have to give much conscious thought to or actively work on. It's a cool process that you once went through that lets you focus on more important shit than food worry and body hate. That doesn't mean you don't check in once in a while, but it's mostly to remind yourself of what an absolute shit show diet culture is. Just to be clear – there's no big graduation party at the end of this process. There are no before-and-after pictures, there's no certificate for 'biggest loser', and if anyone does comment on your body, you feel like telling them where to go. Intuitive eating just becomes a regular part of life. Sorry!

ARE YOU AN INTUITIVE EATER?

Intuitive eating is fundamentally a self-care practice – that means doing what feels helpful and supportive for you (and binning the rest). Therefore, in many ways intuitive eating is subjective – there's no right or wrong, there's only getting in touch with what feels good to you. That said, for research purposes, scientists have developed an intuitive eating assessment called the Intuitive Eating Scale 2 (because it's the second iteration).[18] This tool is used in a lot of research on intuitive eating as a way for researchers to understand how it relates to other things, like body image, mood, and physical health. I'm including an adapted version here, not because there's one 'right' way to do intuitive eating, but more so you can find out about where you're at right now.

The quiz

Read the questions below and check the box next to the ones you agree with. For each check mark, give yourself 1 point, then tally up your score at the end of each section.

1

Unconditional permission to eat

- ☑ I try to avoid certain foods high in fat, carbs, sugar, or kcals
- ☑ I have forbidden foods that I don't let myself eat
- ☑ I get mad at myself for eating something unhealthy
- ☐ If I crave a certain food, I don't allow myself to have it
- ☑ I follow rules that dictate what/when/how much to eat

Score 4 / 5

2

Eating for physical rather than emotional reasons

Even though I'm not physically hungry, I eat when I'm feeling . . .
- ☑ Emotional (anxious, depressed, sad)
- ☑ Lonely
- ☑ Bored
- ☐ Stressed out
- ☑ I use food to help me soothe negative emotions

Score _5_ / 5

3

Reliance on hunger and satiety cues

- ☑ I don't trust my body to tell me when to eat
- ☑ I don't trust my body to tell me what to eat
- ☑ I don't trust my body to tell me how much to eat
- ☑ I don't trust my body to tell me when to stop eating
- ☐ I can't tell when I'm slightly hungry
- ☑ I can't tell when I'm slightly full

Score _5_ / 6

4

Body–food choice congruence

- ☐ Most of the time, I don't want to eat nutritious foods
- ☑ I don't often eat foods that make my body perform well
- ☑ I don't often eat foods that give my body energy and stamina

Score _2_ / 3

Total Score _16_ / 19

In your journal, make a note of the answers to the following questions

+ Which area(s) did you get the highest score in? *All of them*

+ Which area(s) did you get the lowest score in? *None*

+ Did any of these results surprise you? *No*

+ Did any of them really resonate with you? *Yes*

In this adapted version, the lower your score, the more of an intuitive eater you are. If your score is high, please don't freak out: it doesn't mean things are hopeless or you're a lost cause! Besides, although the quiz can be useful to revisit from time to time as you're working through the book, and will give you some insight into areas you might want to think more about, it's not a perfect tool. The concepts are more nuanced than the quiz allows for and we're not aiming for perfection with these scores. In fact, if you are coming out with *perfect* scores (0s for everything), I'd be a bit suspicious. For instance, I've noticed that clients who are very, very rigid and restrictive and may even have anorexia nervosa tend to score highly on *eating for physical rather than emotional needs*. This isn't because they have this aspect of intuitive eating nailed, but because they tend to be really inflexible with their eating; they might not even be eating for physical reasons, let alone emotional ones. So be careful how you interpret this quiz and use it to be curious about your experience, rather than as something to 'get right'; it's only one aspect of tracking our progress, not the final word.

Interpreting your results

You might have noticed that this quiz had four sections to it: *unconditional permission to eat, eating for physical rather than emotional reasons, reliance on hunger and satiety cues, and body–food choice congruence.* The researchers have distilled what we've listed as the ten principles into just four sections for the quiz, representing the four underlying constituent parts, which can also be described as the most common characteristics of intuitive eaters. Let's try and understand these in a little more detail.

Unconditional permission to eat: This is a difficult concept for people to get their heads around. It's essentially the opposite of all the rules, rigidity, and restrictions of dietland. But something that's important to understand is that just because we have *permission* to eat all of the food, doesn't mean we *will* eat all of the food. Nobody is stopping you from quitting your job and going to California, but you probably won't. You have permission to sack off your laundry and just buy new underwear every week; I'm guessing you don't typically do that either. Chances are, you've gone down that path a little way and realized there are consequences. You'd spend all your money on underwear, or realize you need a job to be able to fund your Cali lifestyle. Nobody enforced these 'rules'; you figured them out on your own. This ability to figure out rules on our own is called a *natural contingency* in psychology.[19] Psychologists believe that if our lives are dictated by excessive rules that have been externally imposed on us (and then reinforced by the critical voice in our minds), this leads to human suffering. If we have blanket rules about things, there's no space for us to figure out what works for us in any given context.

Know what has a whole bunch of rules? *Diets*. And because they've been imposed on us from outside (i.e. diet culture), we never have the opportunity to learn flexibility when it comes to eating. When we are little, we might have more natural contingency around tuning into hunger and fullness cues, and less noise from diet culture. But as we grow into adults, natural contingency is replaced by increasingly complex rules, restrictions, 'shoulds' and 'shouldn'ts' and 'musts' (hilariously known as 'must-erbation').

So unconditional permission to eat is simply an invitation to learn what flexible eating looks and feels like for us. We may think

[handwritten margin note: how does this relate to a life of faith?]

it's a cool idea to eat doughnuts all day, but the reality is that after one or two doughnuts we've probably had enough and eating them all day long wouldn't feel great in our bodies. The reason we know that though is through learning and discovering ourselves, a natural contingency, rather than through elaborate rules created by diet culture and reinforced by our judgey brain.

Reliance on hunger and satiety cues: In the same way as we learn a whole bunch of diet rules from diet culture, we also learn that our innate hunger and fullness cues are unreliable. Even as little kids we're taught not to trust the information our bodies are communicating. Well-intentioned messages to 'finish your plate' before going out to play, or 'you can't be hungry AGAIN', serve to undermine what we're innately in tune with. And then as adults, we are taught elaborate schemes to keep hunger at bay. Or to override our body's cues in favour of calories, points or carbs. It's easy to see how the trust in our internal body cues gets replaced with external cues for eating; psychological, emotional, and social cues replace what's going on inside. Reliance on hunger and satiety cues doesn't mean we don't pay attention to those other cues, just that they are integrated with our body's cues. For instance, sometimes after exercise or when we're anxious about stuff, we might not feel much physical hunger, but we know it's important to eat to nourish ourselves. Other times we may have only eaten thirty minutes ago, but our bellies are telling us we're still hungry and need to grab a snack.

Eating for physical rather than emotional reasons: This also requires a more nuanced explanation. We're going to get into this way more down the line, but for now it's important to understand that there's nothing inherently wrong with using food to comfort ourselves – I will be the first person to admit that I turn to comforting foods when things are tough. The difficulty comes when food becomes our only coping mechanism. Later on, we'll talk about how

HOW TO JUST EAT IT

to build up our intuitive eating toolkit so we have a variety of things to choose from to help us deal with the hard shit; if you decide that chocolate is the most helpful tool for a given problem, then that's cool too. The important point is that it was a conscious choice rather than your only choice.

Body–food choice congruence: This relates to how closely our food choices meet our physical and emotional needs. It's not about eating 'perfectly', or only making the most nutritious choices. It's learning that foods that are nutritious are also tasty and satisfying. It's being curious about our physical and emotional needs and learning to honour them through noticing how they make us feel throughout our bodies.

HOW DO WE MEASURE PROGRESS IN INTUITIVE EATING?

So if the IES-2 is only one metric of progress, how do we know how we're doing? Unlike diets, there's no finish line with intuitive eating; we don't count calories, carbs, or kilos lost. There's no measuring your waist or hips or checking clothes sizes. These are all external metrics of 'success', but intuitive eating is an internal process. It's also not a diet and the goal is not weight loss, so we have to change what progress means. In fact, I don't really even like using the terms 'progress' or 'success'; they feel very diet-y to me and reinforce the problematic capitalist notion that we constantly have to be striving for self-improvement at all costs. Now, don't get me wrong, I think it's great to be learning new skills and growing as humans, but if that isn't coming from a place of acceptance and self-compassion, it ends up being a tool for distraction and disconnection. From this perspective, we need to shift our perception of what progress means in the context of intuitive eating.

Diets and attempts to shrink our body are usually coming from a place of disliking ourselves and are accompanied by a narrative of how much better we will be, or our lives will be, once we lose X amount of weight. This is the fundamental lie of diet culture; there is no pot of gold at the end of the rainbow, so we keep chasing ever more unrealistic and unrelenting beauty and body standards to feel OK about ourselves. So how can we keep tabs on what happens when we move through the intuitive eating process? Well, like I said, it's an internal shift, so we need to be reflecting and looking inwards to notice what's going on, with curiosity and non-judgement. This might look like:

* Shifts in our self-talk – less trash-talking ourselves and our bodies.

* Eating in response to physical cues instead of suppressing or ignoring them.

* Noticing ourselves being more self-compassionate.

* More flexibility in our approach to food – less dichotomizing food as 'good' or 'bad'.

* Taking more pleasure and satisfaction from food.

* Dedicating less headspace to thoughts of food, diets, weight, and exercise.

* Being kinder to our bodies.

* Asking ourselves what kind of movement might feel good and give us joy.

* Being curious about where our desire to lose weight is coming from rather than just acting on it.

* Feeling less apprehensive or fearful of social situations involving food.

* Engaging more fully in areas of life that are fulfilling and life-enhancing.

Some people will measure 'success' in terms of behaviours – less bingeing or 'emotional' eating, for example. While these are important too, try and notice the internal shifts that give rise to these changes in behaviour. At the end of each section, there's an opportunity to reflect on any shifts you've noticed along the way.

In your journal, write down what intuitive eating looks like for you

What does intuitive eating mean to you?

Before we move on with the nuts and bolts of intuitive eating, it's helpful to define what exactly it is we're working towards, and what we want to get out of the process.

Think about how it would feel to be an intuitive eater. How would you know you were eating intuitively? Would you think about food a little or a lot? Would eating be flexible or rigid? If your friend invited you out for an impromptu pizza, would you be able to accept their invite without freaking out? What does your self-talk around food sound like? Are you able to show yourself more compassion, particularly when things get bumpy? Can you tune into your body's own cues, paying attention to early-warning signs of hunger and sensing when your energy levels dip? Are you eating a wider variety of foods (including fun foods)? What does your self-care look like? Can you honour your body's need for both rest and movement? If you're an intuitive eater, does it open up more space to pursue opportunities in other areas of your life? What does it allow you to do?

Of course, your answers might change over time as you learn new skills and deepen your understanding of what IE is. It can be helpful to return periodically to check in with yourself.

* eating mostly fresh + in season
* enjoying food
* thinking about food when I am hungry
* not bingeing
* doing a range of self-care activities when I want to self-comfort —AND— dealing directly w/ those situations

HOW TO JUST EAT IT

* spending less on food
* eating at home / trying new recipes

YOUR RESEARCH

So, as promised, I'm not going to spoon-feed you; I'm going to ask you to do some research of your own! Intuitive eating is a process of discovery, both learning about what is right for you and your body (on your terms), but also an education in all the broader concepts that underpin the intuitive eating framework. The anti-diet movement was born out of body liberation and justice for all bodies, and when we work on intuitive eating, we need to hold in mind that the implications are far wider-reaching than for us as individuals. For intuitive eating to 'click' as a personal practice, it helps to have a good grounding in the theory as well as the practice. We'll return to these ideas throughout the book and will look at them more closely in the last section, Chapter 12 – Where We Go From Here.

Glossary

Listen to the podcast episode for this section (*Introduction*) and check out the resources named below to help you come up with definitions in your journal for each of the terms listed on page 36. Each of these are big topics and it's worthwhile taking your time to dig deep and make sure you understand them. You'll also find definitions throughout the podcast.

Don't Salt My Game – How to Just Eat It: various

* The Anti-Diet Project on Refinery 29

* Christy Harrison's blog and podcast (Food Psych)

* Virgie Tovar's blog on Forbes.com

* YourFatFriend.com

* Regan Chastain's blog DancesWithFat.org

* 'Poodle Science' by ASDAH on YouTube

* She's All Fat podcast

* GenerousPlan.com

* My Black Body Podcast

Some of these concepts might be totally foreign to you; they might also make you feel uncomfortable. That's OK – try and work through the discomfort; it's just a sign that you're learning and growing.

Anti-diet	Health at Every Size
Body liberation	Healthism
Body neutrality	Intersectional feminism
Body positivity (or BoPo)	Marginalization
Diet culture	Pseudo-diet
Disordered eating	Privilege
Eating disorders*	Social determinants of health
Fat activism	Thin/size privilege
Fat phobia	The thin ideal
Fitspo	Weight bias vs weight stigma

* anorexia, orthorexia, binge-eating disorder and bulimia nervosa are the 'major' categories – note that these can occur in people of all body shapes and sizes

Why Diet Culture Sucks

Artika Gunathasan
BOPO, fitness and mental
health advocate
@arti.speaks

When you hear the phrase 'diet culture', you'd be forgiven for thinking it all started with tabloid magazines tearing down curvier women with cellulite, those Pinterest articles on foods that help you 'burn fat' (not a thing), and celebrities being paid to promote 'detox' teas and powders that are essentially overpriced laxatives (and can sometimes mess with your contraceptive pill). We think of diet culture as something that began within our lifetime, invented by whatever media we consumed from our childhood or early teens. The truth is that diet culture has been deeply ingrained in our society far longer than that.

Diet culture is rooted in sexist and racist oppression, and further perpetuates the policing and othering of poor, disabled, and queer bodies. It's an uncomfortable truth, but acknowledging this fact can help us escape the destructive cycle of restricting and self-loathing as we contribute to a multi-billion-dollar industry that doesn't serve us at all.

The beginnings of fat phobia and dieting can be traced back to the transatlantic slave trade when, in the early 1800s, white colonialists perpetuated the idea that larger Black bodies were the result of laziness and gluttony. White women were encouraged to pursue thinness – a marker of white superiority – at least 100 years before medical establishments began discussing 'excess' weight and its potential health implications. This divisive tactic birthed a narrative fuelled by modern-day capitalism that placed higher value on figures that appear thin and able-bodied – and thus able to form a more reliable workforce – while people in larger bodies and those with disabilities were further dehumanized, viewed as having a poorer work ethic and therefore more disposable.

Over the course of the last 200 years, diet culture has evolved to affect people of all backgrounds and body sizes, by encouraging everyone to attain body standards that are mostly unattainable without negatively affecting other aspects of our lives. Very few people benefit from this.

Women's bodies are viewed through trends, like the 1920s flapper or the curvaceous Instagram baddie; and not fitting these moulds leads to body image issues and chauvinism. Narrow body ideals in queer culture contribute to the higher prevalence of eating disorders in gay and bisexual men compared to heterosexual men. Diet culture and fat phobia fuel body image issues in trans folk who already face discrimination for not conforming to patriarchal gender (binary) norms. Black, Brown, and Indigenous people see their cultural dishes misappropriated through the lens of diet culture, as they are reduced and demonized through the weaponization of Western food science.

Diet culture can leave people with certain physical disabilities feeling further excluded in an already ableist society. Like the other aforementioned marginalized groups, there is pressure to assimilate to an unattainable standard, and this becomes an even steeper uphill climb when there are barriers to a person's access to suitable food, exercise, and side effect-free medication. Folks with larger bodies face weight stigma that impacts their mental health, relationships, how they are treated by their doctor, and even their job prospects – as they are presumed to be unhealthy and lazy. Diet culture also encourages the vilification of working-class people and people in the underclass, who have limited access to food and health choices and are, like larger people, slammed for being lazy and asking for handouts.

This is just a brief rundown of a handful of ways that diet culture makes life harder for everyone, but in particular for marginalized groups. People who hold intersecting identities endure even more complex negative experiences. Abandoning and eradicating diet culture won't erase these issues, as they stem from historically oppressive systems that are yet to be dismantled.

So why abandon diet culture at all? Speaking as a Diet Culture Dropout, it has been a blessing. Not only has my relationship with food improved in general, the fact that I don't have food rules surrounding what and how often I can eat means that I don't compulsively eat or secretively eat 'banned' food. I experience much less anxiety and guilt over food, particularly during celebrations when food has a lot of cultural importance. I rarely think about needing to 'work off' food through the exercise that I do; and I am able to view exercise as a form of joyful movement. My body image is so much better and I am better able to explore body neutrality and detach my self-worth from my body shape or size.

Looking back, and consuming media that is still very diet- and thin-centric with a new world view, I am amazed that I didn't realize how fucked up the messaging and impact of this narrative is: that we need to obey the food police and strive to perfect our bodies over and over, despite 'failing' and 'falling off the wagon' over and over – through no fault of our own (although that's not what we're led to believe). It genuinely feels as though society has normalized the masses into coercing ourselves and each other into conforming, or face being ostracized.

Let's stop bullying ourselves. Let's give ourselves more kindness, more love, and more permission to eat what we want. Let's drop out of diet culture.

In your journal, make a note of the answers to the following questions

➕ What in the intuitive eating process are you most excited about? *freedom from food + fear of man in relation to my size + diet*

➕ What do you think might be more challenging for you? *emotional eating - letting go of losing weight*

➕ How can you be kind and gentle to yourself in the more challenging moments? *focus on self-care and addressing negative self-talk*

➕ How can you celebrate the little light bulbs coming on along the way? *journal regularly + be present so I am able to notice both the "big" + "little" areas of growth in thoughts + actions*

CHAPTER 1

LAYING THE FOUNDATION

Your Intuitive Eating Toolkit

Listen to the corresponding podcast episode Don't Salt My Game – How to Just Eat It: Chapter 1

It's tempting to want to go hard or go home with this intuitive eating stuff. Look, I get it! After years of hopping on and off the dieting merry-go-round, you probably want to get the hell out of dietland and never look back. And while I love your motivation, I want to set you up with a really solid foundation for building your intuitive eating skills on. That means creating a toolkit that helps you navigate the process with intention, compassion, and kindness. In this section, I'm sharing some of the tools clients find most useful, but I'm guessing you already have a few of your own that you can add in. The bulk of the tools are in this section, but there are plenty more throughout the book; come back and add to your toolkit each time you come across one that you find helpful. By having all of your tools in one place, you'll be better equipped to deal with difficulties and challenges that pop up – like having to deal with fat-phobic relatives at Christmas parties or office diet talk. Clients have also shared with me that having these tools doesn't just make the IE process easier, but helps them deal with other life stuff too. That's one of the cool things about intuitive eating: we're learning these skills in the microcosm of our relationship to food and our bodies, but the impact is so much bigger than that.

> This section is suitable for people with active eating disorders. There are a bunch of tools and skills contained here that will help support your eating disorder recovery

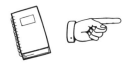

Building your own toolkit

As you move through the book, write down the tools, skills, and coping strategies you have developed that help you deal with the tough stuff that life throws at you. Some folks prefer to make a physical version of their toolkit – a wooden or cardboard box to put physical tools in (aromatherapy oils, stress ball, etc), as well as physical representations of the tools discussed here. Maybe that's drawing a picture of the sushi train (page 52), or practising some written defusion techniques (page 48). It's your toolkit, so do whatever makes it feel supportive and accessible to you.

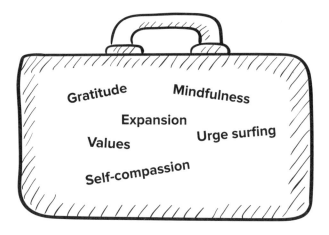

Add any existing tools you have to your toolkit and keep adding new ones as you move through the book

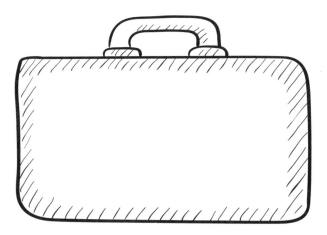

GROUNDING

Grounding is a technique whereby we calm our nervous system, so we feel physically and emotionally centred. I like to think of it as the earth wire in a plug; it helps diffuse electricity, so it doesn't overload a system. We can use grounding techniques to soothe ourselves when we feel anxious, stressed, or nervous. It can be equally useful when we're overly excited or stimulated and need to focus.

Anchoring

Anchoring, or 'dropping anchor', is a great metaphor for navigating emotions. Just like the weather, emotions can be calm and clear like on a fine day. On other days it might be a bit overcast, and on yet other days there can be a full-blown storm. When the weather gets rough, ships need a harbour, so they'll drop an anchor to help keep them steady as they ride out the storm; it doesn't change the weather, but it keeps the ship safe and secure. Humans can drop metaphorical anchors when things feel overwhelming or bumpy, but it helps to practise when the weather is clear, so that when a storm hits, we know exactly what we need to do. Anchoring has three main components.

The following is adapted from *Act Mindfully*[1]

Noticing and naming thoughts and feelings: When we are having a tough time, we naturally want to escape from difficult feelings. However, trying to push them down, avoid, or ignore them doesn't actually help us release them; instead they get stuck and can end up manifesting physically or popping up in unwanted places, like a never-ending game of whack-a-mole. By turning towards and acknowledging difficult feelings, we can help them flow through us more easily. This won't necessarily make them go away, but they might feel a little less powerful, particularly if you combine noticing and naming with the other elements of anchoring.

Add to the list any other ways you've found to help you tune into your body

Grounding into your body: The second aspect of anchoring is to tune into your physical body. It sounds counterintuitive, but if you get stuck in your mind about negative body image thoughts, then actually sinking *into* your body can be really powerful. Take a few moments to practise a few of the following methods. Try and be intentional and deliberate about each one, focusing on the sensations in your body as you do the actions.

* Touching your fingertips together with your thumb, one by one from index to pinky and back again Repeat several times.

* Sitting up tall, push the soles of your feet into the ground. Feel the firm ground beneath you and notice you are safe.

* Stretch your arms out in all directions. Really feel all the way into your fingertips. Hold for a few seconds, feeling a good stretch in your arms and along your back.

* Standing or sitting, allow your torso to sway side to side. Feel the movement of your rib cage; your head might even come along for the ride. Notice if this helps you release tension.

* Sitting or standing, gently twist your torso to the right and then to the left (like you might in a yoga class, being careful not to overstretch). Hold each side for a few seconds.

* Clasp your hands behind your back and gently stretch them downwards, feeling a light tugging sensation all the way down your arms into your wrists.

* Nod your chin down towards your chest and lightly roll or tilt your head from side to side, feeling a stretch in your neck.

* ....

* ....

* ....

Connecting with the physical space: A bit like grounding into your body, connecting with the physical space reminds us that we are OK and helps us feel less 'in our heads'. There are loads of ways to do this – experiment and find what works best for you. Again, try not to blast through this, but take some time connecting with each one.

Add to the list any other ways you've found to help you tune into your body

* Name five things you can see, touch four objects around you, notice three sounds (nearby or in the distance), notice two smells (could be perfume, laundry detergent, or a yucky bin close by!), notice one taste in your mouth (toothpaste, coffee, the remnants of lunch).

* Name as many different colours in the room as you can see.

* Reach out and stroke a pet, noticing the texture of their fur/ skin, the temperature, the relative softness or coarseness of their hair.

* Run your hands under cool water for a few moments, noticing how the water flows around your palms and fingers.

* Wrap yourself in a warm blanket or place a hot water bottle on your lap.

* Smell some essential oils or an aromatherapy candle.

* Gently squeeze a stress ball or some Play-Doh.

* ....

* ....

* ....

If it's helpful, record in your journal which methods work best for you the next few times you practise this technique, using the following headings. The more you practise it in a structured way, the more easily you'll be able to tap into it in moments of difficulty

Now combine these three components for the complete practice: notice and name the uncomfortable thought or feeling, ground down into your body, and connect with the physical space you're in. Repeat this process as many times as you need to until you feel you have soothed and comforted yourself. Like I said, it helps massively to practise this when the weather is calm, so that when the seas inevitably get choppier, you know what to do.

* Notice and name what I'm feeling.

* Physical practices to help ground me in my body.

* Connect with the physical space – what did I notice?

Repeat the above steps as many times as needed.

DEFUSION

Have you ever noticed a thought so strong and urgent that it felt like a command? Like if you didn't do exactly as it said, something terrible would happen? This can often arise in relation to food and dieting rules we've internalized over time. They might sound a bit like this:

Technique adapted from *ACT Made Simple*[2]

'If you eat that cookie, it will blow your diet'

'Gaining weight makes you worthless'

'You need to go to the gym, you fat, lazy slob'

'My thighs are huge'

These thoughts can feel powerful and overwhelming, like little bombs going off in our brain. But it doesn't mean they are true. And just like bombs, we can learn to defuse them. OK, maybe you aren't defusing a bomb in your day-to-day life, but you get the idea. We can neutralize our thoughts by learning to observe them, rather than automatically buying into them. Let's try something to help illustrate what I mean.

Step 1: Write down a difficult thought

Identify a food- or body-related thought that comes up all the time. Something that seems to play on a loop in your mind. Pick something upsetting but not distressing. Note it down in your journal.

Step 2: Record and listen

Record the following passage on your phone and play it back to yourself. It asks you to cover your eyes with your hands, so you can't read it while doing the activity!

Sitting somewhere quietly and comfortably where you won't be disturbed, notice the space in the room around you . . . Imagine that space is filled with all the things you care about: people you love, things you're passionate about, your achievements and accomplishments, cats and dogs, maybe your favourite artists, nature . . . All the stuff that makes you get out of bed in the morning . . . Really take the time to notice all these things . . .

Now, also notice the room is filled with the difficulties and challenges you have . . . the things that you're struggling with . . . and the things you wish could be different . . .

Notice that ALL that stuff is there, the positive, the negative, and the somewhere-in-between stuff . . .

Now, holding your hands out in front of you, like the pages of a book, imagine that negative thought from earlier written a thousand times over. Play it in your mind a few times . . . this should feel uncomfortable, but not overwhelmingly so . . . Notice how it feels to be hooked into that thought, to really believe it's true . . . Notice how we let that thought pull us in different directions . . . a simple thought can become a whole story . . .

When you feel bought into that thought, slowly bring your hands up to your eyes and cover them completely . . . Repeat the thought a few times over . . .

Now, with your eyes covered, notice what it feels like to engage with all the things in the space around you . . . all the things you value and care about . . . How easy is it to connect with loved ones? How easy is it to deal with the tough stuff? What does it feel like with those words really in your face . . . How easy is it to breathe? Does it feel claustrophobic? Spend a moment sitting with these feelings . . .

Now, slowly and gently bring your hands away from your face . . . maybe 10cm or so. Notice how it feels when you make a little space . . . Does it become easier to connect with the space around you? Is it easier to breathe?

Now let your hands fall into your lap . . . How does this feel?

Step 3: Write down your feelings

* How did it feel to have your hands up covering your eyes? Claustrophobic, upsetting, disconnected, unsettling, difficult to engage with the world?

* How did it feel to bring your hands down from your face? Created space, easier to breathe, better able to deal with the tough stuff?

Bringing our hands down away from our face represents what it's like when we defuse our difficult thoughts. Notice that your hands didn't go anywhere, they were still there; you just had some distance from them. It's the same with our thoughts. Sure, we can try and argue with them and rationalize, but that doesn't always help, and sometimes makes things worse. What we can do instead is to notice what happens when we *observe* our thoughts and get *curious* about them, instead of judging them or getting sucked into them. I want to stress here that these exercises are not intended for defusing important thoughts that impact your safety or well-being. For instance, being fused to the thought that 'a car is heading towards me' is probably an important one that we want to pay attention to so we can get out of the road. Likewise, if you're fused to the storyline of a movie or a book you're reading, that has value for your life. The 'I'm gross and disgusting' narrative that plays on loop? Not so much. It gets in the way of creating meaning and purpose. So how can we notice that it's there, but not let it take us on a ride? The exercises in this section will help you learn more skills around this.

> ### Defusion practice
>
> Remember, the intention is not to get rid of thoughts or a particular feeling associated with these thoughts (like anxiety), but to see if we can learn not to take our thoughts quite so seriously, particularly the ones that aren't actually helpful or useful. Also, the key is to practise. Many clients tell me that these techniques can be helpful, but they need to repeat them a few times over in order to be able to use them in a difficult moment.

Try practising the following defusion techniques, either in your head or aloud

I AM NOTICING THAT . . .

* Recall the difficult thought you had earlier. Now repeat it to yourself five or six times over. Really *feel* what it's like when you speak that way to yourself.

* Now say 'I am noticing that . . .' in front of the thought. Repeat it a few times over.

* Now say 'I am noticing that I'm having the thought that . . .' in front of the thought. Practise saying the whole thing a few times over. 'I am noticing that I'm having the thought that . . .', 'I am noticing that I'm having the thought that . . .', 'I am noticing that I'm having the thought that . . .'

　　　　HOW TO JUST EAT IT

> Notice how it feels. Is it any easier to take the thought less seriously? Does it feel any less threatening? Does it help open up some space?

SING THE THOUGHT

Try singing the thought to the tune of a classic like 'Happy Birthday', 'Jingle Bells', 'Twinkle Twinkle Little Star' or whatever your favourite tune is.

In clinic, I make people sing their thought out loud. People understandably feel a bit shy about it. But after we've both sung a couple of lines of 'my thighs are too big' to the tune of 'Jingle Bells', we can usually laugh about it. It doesn't make the thought go away, but it can help it sting a little less.

> How did it feel singing the words out loud? Did it help open up a little bit of space where you could take the thought less seriously? Did it at least make you laugh a little?

IN THE VOICE OF

Another cute technique for defusion is saying the thought aloud in the distinctive voice of a famous person. Like the singing example above, saying it out loud has more impact. My husband makes me do this whenever I get trolling comments on my Instagram account. I say them in a funny voice, and instantly it helps me see it's their shit, not mine. I can then respond a little more gracefully. It can be literally any voice you like, but here are some ideas.

Add your own to this list!

* Janice from *Friends*

* Jonathan Van Ness (try saying anything mean about yourself in a JVN voice – I DARE YOU)

* Homer Simpson

* ....

* ....

* ....

> How did it feel saying the words in a different voice? Did it help you unhook from the thoughts, even for just a moment?

Advanced defusion – the sushi train

The tools I shared above are great in a pickle – you can imagine bringing your hands down from your face as you practice any of the above techniques. I think you might just about be ready to kick it up a level, but before we start, I have a question for you. However, I don't want you to answer straight away. Once I ask it, I want you to wait ten seconds before writing down the answer. A full ten seconds. Don't cheat. Ready? OK!

Q: Knock knock?
A:

Did you write 'Who's there?' I bet you did. And I bet it was really tough not to write it down straight away instead of waiting for ten seconds. I hope you did wait though, because there's an important lesson in here. Did you notice that your mind answered the question in a split second? You almost immediately came up with the answer. But then another part of your mind said 'Hit the brakes, we have to wait ten seconds', and then maybe it started counting down. This example helps us illustrate two parts of our brain. A reflexive, automatic part of our brain that acts on instinct and impulse – we can call this the *automatic mind*. Then there's a calmer and more measured part of our brain that notices what the automatic mind is up to. This is our *observer mind*. Now, to be clear, this doesn't mean there's a 'good' and 'bad' part of our brain. Our automatic mind serves an important function – like getting our ass out of the road when there's a car coming! – but the observer mind acts as an important balance, helping prevent us from getting carried away by the automatic mind when it's not being helpful, as is often the case when we are body-bashing or letting food rules call the shots. Keep this in mind as we talk about the sushi train.

THE SUSHI TRAIN

Imagine yourself in one of those sushi restaurants that has a conveyor belt of plates circling around it. In the middle of the restaurant is a sushi chef, prepping all the dishes and stacking the plates onto the conveyor belt. Next to him is an empty stack of plates, all ready and waiting for something to be plated up and passed onto the conveyor belt. You are sitting in the restaurant, watching the sushi pass by. (Don't worry if you don't like sushi; you can imagine any sort of food you want on the plates themselves – just try and get the visual.) OK, now start to notice the contents of the plates as they make their way around the restaurant. There are some plates you like, find satisfying and pleasant, that bring you pleasure, maybe like a salmon sashimi. There are some plates you could sort of take or leave – these are foods you feel pretty neutral about, like a cucumber roll. They'll fill you up and they keep you going, but they're nothing out of the ordinary or all that special, but they're basically just fuel. And

Adapted from
Reyelle-McKeever[3]

there are some plates you wouldn't eat even if someone paid you, something that's gone off and is rotten, maybe? The chef is in charge of which plates come out and when. Sometimes there's a spate of sashimi, sometimes it's a run of rotten plates, but most of the time it's just cucumber roll. You are in charge of which plates you pick up and which ones you let go by.

The sushi chef is like our automatic mind: they decide which plates of food go out, in which order, just like the thoughts our automatic mind generates (which are often critical and judgemental). You, sitting in the restaurant, watching the plates pass by, are like the observing mind – that part of our brain that can watch thoughts float past, without necessarily acting on every single one. In other words, you get to decide which plates you pick up and which you leave on the train. It wouldn't make sense if you were to pick up all the rotten plates, right? You'd have to pay for something you either didn't eat, or that made you feel sick and gross.

Now let's start putting your plates on the sushi train.

* What is a plate you'd find really tasty that you'd definitely want to pick up off the *sushi train*? (It doesn't have to be sushi, but could be pizza or croissants or anything else you like.)

* What does this plate represent in terms of your *train of thought*? (For example, 'I feel a sense of pride over X accomplishment'. Or 'I am a genuinely caring friend'.)

* What is a plate you feel neutral about that you could take or leave on the *sushi train*? (For instance, cherry tomatoes or popcorn.)

* What does this plate represent in terms of your *train of thought*? (For instance, 'the weather is a bit shit', 'I need to remember to do the washing'.)

* Lastly, what is a plate you find really repulsive and disgusting that you wouldn't want to pick up from *the sushi train*? (Think

of something really horrible, something rotten, something you're allergic to or your least favourite food.)

✳ What does this plate represent in terms of your *train of thought*? (It could be something you've already picked out, but anything critical or judgemental around food and body would work.)

I'm going to take a guess that you probably picked up a lot of that last kind of plate from the sushi train. Even though you don't like it or want it. In the same way, we have a tendency to buy into thoughts and stories that our automatic mind is churning out that don't really serve us. But just like the 'sushi restaurant you', your observing mind can sit back and notice these thoughts without acting on them.

So what could you do if you were to accidentally pick up a plate of bad sushi that you didn't want? Well, you could push it to the side and try to ignore it, but ultimately it would still be sitting there, stinking up the place. Another option might be to put it back on the sushi train. Unlike the sushi train, the train in our minds isn't a closed loop. We can opt to put the bad sushi back on the train, and watch them drift away, ultimately falling off the end of the conveyor. In this sense, we are also defusing those thoughts.

> Notice when you are experiencing 'bad sushi' thoughts. Can you acknowledge they are there but let them pass by? If you do accidentally pick some up, can you practice putting them back on the conveyor belt?

EXPANSION

Expansion is a technique for helping you sit with difficult or uncomfortable emotions and feelings instead of getting caught in a battle with them. Often when we experience something uncomfortable, we engage in a struggle with it, trying to push it down or wish it away. This can end up making things worse and can be ultimately self-defeating. The goal here isn't to get rid of the feeling – that would be a form of emotional avoidance – but to become familiar with it and begin to understand what it's communicating to you.

Again, you might want to record this on your phone so you can play it back to yourself (or get a friend or family member to record it for you)

Expansion practice

STEP 1: OBSERVE THE SENSATIONS IN YOUR BODY

Start by taking a few deeps breaths . . . breathing in through your nose . . . and out through your mouth . . . In through your nose, and out through your mouth . . . and once more, breathing in through the nose and out through the mouth. Take a few seconds to scan yourself from your head to your toes. As you do this, you will probably notice several uncomfortable sensations. Look for the one that bothers you the most. For example, it may be a lump in your throat, a knot in your stomach, anxiety in your chest, or a teary feeling in your eyes. Now focus your attention on that sensation. Observe it with curiosity, like a scientist who has discovered some interesting new phenomenon. Notice where it starts and where it stops. If you had to draw an outline around this sensation, what shape would it have? Is it on the surface of the body, or inside you, or both? How far inside you does it go? Where is it most intense? Where is it weakest? How is it different in the centre from around the edges? Is there any pulse or vibration? Is it light or heavy? Warm or cool? Moving or still? What colour is it? Does it have any textures or patterns? Is it heavy or light?

STEP 2: BREATHE

Breathe into and around the sensation. Begin with a few deep breaths (the slower the better) and make sure you empty your lungs fully as you breathe out. Slow, deep breathing is important because it helps you lower the levels of tension in your body. It won't get rid of your feelings, but it will provide a centre of calm within you. It's like an anchor in the midst of a storm. It won't get rid of the storm, but it will hold you steady until it passes. So breathe deeply and slowly, and imagine your breath flowing into and around the sensation.

STEP 3: CREATE SPACE

As your breath flows into and around the sensation or feeling, it's as if you are somehow creating extra space within your body. You open up and create a space around this sensation, giving it plenty of room to move. And if it gets bigger, you give it even more space. Take a few more deep breaths, in through your nose and out through your mouth. In through your nose, and out through your mouth, in through your nose and out through your mouth, creating more space with each breath.

STEP 4: ALLOW

Allow the sensation to be there, even though you don't like it or want it. In other words, just let it be. When your mind starts commenting on what's happening, say, 'thanks for the story, mind' and come back to observing the sensation. Of course, you might find this difficult and feel a strong urge to fight with this feeling, or push it away. If so, just acknowledge the urge. You can even imagine yourself nodding in

Adapted from
The Happiness Trap
by Russ Harris[4]

recognition of the urge, saying to yourself, 'there you are; I see you'.
Then, very gently, bring your attention back to the sensation itself.

Remember the intention here is not to get rid of the sensation or alter it. It may change on its own and that's OK. Equally it may not change at all, and that's also OK. Changing or getting rid of the sensation is not the goal here. The goal is to make space for it, to allow it to flow through you without getting stuck, to make peace with it, and to let it be, even if you don't like it or want it.

You may need some more time to focus on the sensation before you can give up the struggle with it. Be patient and take as long as you need. You can practise alone, or listen to this meditation again to remind yourself of the steps. Practise as often as needed and feel free to repeat this activity for any other unpleasant sensations you might be experiencing.

In your journal, make a note of the answers to the following questions

+ What sensation did you notice?

+ Where was it?

+ How would you describe it?

+ Can you draw the sensation?

+ How did it feel to observe the sensation and let it move through you?

VALUES

Values are one of my favourite things to discuss with clients, because we all have them, but we rarely slow down and focus in on them. Values describe how we want to move through the world: the type of person we want to be, and how we want to treat others. Unlike goals, values can never be achieved or checked off a list. For instance, if one of your values is kindness, you're not going to be kind just once and then go back to being an asshole. Values are directions we keep moving in that help make our life meaningful, independent of any end goal.

Clarifying our values is helpful when trying to bust out of diet jail because diet culture teaches us to be goals focused: reach a target weight, get our 'best body yet', lift a certain weight, eat a certain (tiny) number of calories. All the parameters of diet culture teach us to strive and achieve something that, sure, might bring us temporary happiness, but will it bring us long-term fulfilment and satisfaction? Chances are that once we hit one goal, we're onto the next one and the one after that. Or we never reach our goal, and we become disappointed and disheartened. We may even stop moving our bodies or eating nutritious foods because we don't see the point; if we can't reach our goal, we don't see the value inherent in those activities. We are conditioned to pursue outcomes and end goals, but we are never given permission to follow a path of fulfilment and joy that may or may not lead anywhere. I've done this activity with loads and loads of clients, and so far nobody has put 'weight loss', 'skinny', or 'counting calories' as values, because at the end of the day, these aren't a reflection of what's truly important to us.

Another way to think about this is admittedly pretty morbid, but I think really hammers home what I mean. I want you to im-agine the eulogy given at your funeral. Yep, you are dead now, and all your friends and family are gathered and they're talking 'bout you. You are now a ghost/spirit/the wind and you can overhear everything that's being said. How do you want those conversations to sound? Are they discussing your commitment to diet culture? 'RIP Debbie, girl could do a lot of sit-ups.' 'Yeah, she was the biggest loser in our slimming group three weeks in a row.' Or do you want to be remembered for the things you stood for, the way you made people feel, and the values you embodied? 'Debbie was such a considerate and loyal friend – I'm going to miss the hell out of her.' 'She really was so much fun to be around; she made people feel so loved and appreciated.'

Write your own epitaph

Using your journal, I'd like you to reflect on what you'd like your life to stand for. What do you want to be remembered for? I know it's super grim, but frankly, a lot of us spend our lives consumed with trying to pursue weight loss, not because it brings us joy and fulfilment, but because we've been told that's how it *should* be. Taking a step back, questioning it and putting some perspective on it can really help remind ourselves what we'd like our lives to stand for. Take your time over this. Don't just write 'I want to be remembered as a good person' – the more specific you can be, the better. Write out how you hope your epitaph will read.

Clarifying your values

Now you've begun to explore what you'd like your life to stand for, we can start homing in on the values driving this. Using the following activity will help you nail them down further.

Using the list below, start to narrow your values down by sorting them into the following categories: important, pretty important, really important, core values. In other words, you will likely have lots of values that are important to you, but we want to get to what's really at the heart of your values. I've noticed that what we think our values are can often be influenced by what we're told our values should be – in other words, our cultural programming – instead of our own authentic set of core values. To get past this, as you are categorizing these values, ask yourself:

* Would this still be a core value for me if nobody could see me do it?

* Would it still be a core value even if it seemed to other people that I was doing something completely different?

* And critically, would this be a core value if it didn't have any impact whatsoever on my body shape or size?

Remember that values are verbs – they're behaviours, not feelings. For example, you may not always feel generous towards people, but can you behave in a generous way?

Acceptance	Connection	Freedom	Learning	Responsibility
Accessibility	Contribution	Friendliness	Liberation	Romance
Adventure	Cooperation	Fun	Love	Safety
Assertiveness	Courage	Generosity	Mindfulness	Self-awareness
Authenticity	Creativity	Gratitude	Non-conformity	Self-care
Beauty	Curiosity	Honesty	Open-mindedness	Sensuality
Benevolence	Discovery	Humility	Passion	Sexuality
Boldness	Encouragement	Humour	Patience	Simplicity
Calmness	Equality	Independence	Peace	Social justice
Caring	Equity	Industry	Persistence	Spirituality
Challenge	Excitement	Inspiration	Play	Stability
Charity	Fairness	Intimacy	Pleasure	Supportiveness
Collaboration	Fearlessness	Joy	Power	Trust
Community	Flexibility	Justice	Reciprocity	
Compassion	Forgiveness	Kindness	Respect	

	Important	Pretty important	Really important	Core values
1				
2				
3				
4				
5				

HOW TO JUST EAT IT

Now you've narrowed it down a little, let's make sure you're super clear on the role values play in your life and what they have to offer. For each of the core values you've selected above, I'd like you to write for *ten minutes* – yes, a full ten minutes. Sounds like a long time, but once you get going it will fly by. You'll probably need to get some additional paper or your journal. Use the following prompts to help guide you.

✷ When in my life have I embodied this value most?

✷ How did I know I was aligned with this value? (What did it look like, feel like, how did I think and act?)

✷ How can I tap into this value more in my life? Would this bring me a sense of fulfilment?

✷ When in my life have I been discordant with this value? Did it cost me anything?

A little note on values – it's important to take care that we are using values to guide direction, fulfilment, and joy in our lives. They're not another tool to get shitty with ourselves about when we think we've fallen short. For instance, maybe one of our core values is compassion, and then we blow up at a friend for a flippant comment they didn't mean. Our reaction probably wasn't very compassionate, but instead of beating ourselves up, can we hold ourselves with compassion and apologize? As Steven Hayes, one of the architects of the ACT model says about values – 'pursue them vigorously but hold them lightly'.

Checking in with your values

Now that we have clarified our core values, we can reflect on how closely we feel we use our values to guide the direction our lives take. Take a moment to reflect on the core values that you feel resonate most with you. Now, using the bullseye illustration below, we can get curious about how congruent or discordant we are with these values in different areas of our lives. This isn't a tool for judgement – we haven't 'failed' if we're more out of touch with our values than we'd like to be – but it offers us an opportunity to tune into what might make us feel more in line with our values more of the time. Take a moment to read about each of the domains below and think about how your core values factor into each – it may not be immediately apparent. For example, it's easy to see how connection might apply to various different relationships, but leisure or well-being might be a bit tougher to figure out. You could consider connection to your body or yourself as being an important part of well-being. Or connection in the sense of being fully present in the moment while at play during leisure activities.

Work: Education, self-directed learning, developing new skills, career.

Spirituality: Organized religion, prayer, worship, meditation, yoga, personal growth, nature.

Family: How you are as a parent, child, sibling, and so on.

Friendships: What is important in your platonic relationships? Think about close friends, colleagues, and acquaintances.

Romantic relationships: The type of partner you want to be and the type of relationship(s) you want to have.

Well-being and personal growth: Mental and physical health and well-being, self-care, medical care, creativity, rest.

Leisure: Recreation, play, relaxation, and enjoyment. Activities that are just for fun and nourish the soul.

Citizenship: Community, activism, volunteering, contributing to a just and fair society.

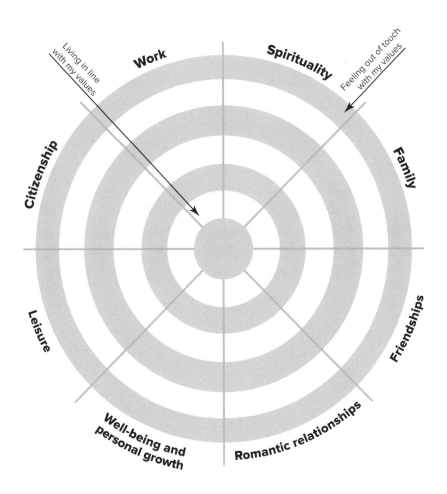

Make a copy of the blank template in the Appendix (see page 309) in your journal. Plot on the bullseye how aligned you feel with your values and notice the areas where you feel less aligned. What are the areas where you feel you are fully living your values? What are the areas where you would like to be more in tune with your values? Make several copies of the blank bullseye so you can fill in a different one for each value.

+ Which tools did you like or connect with most in this section?

+ Have you noticed any fairy lights coming on?

+ Go back to the toolkit section at the beginning of the chapter and start to fill up the blank toolkit with some of the new tools and skills you've learned, along with any you already had.

CHAPTER 2

BREAKING UP WITH DIET CULTURE

Listen to the corresponding podcast episode Don't Salt My Game – How to Just Eat It: Chapter 2

The chances are, you have, at one point or another, been on a diet. You may not have called it a diet: maybe it was a 'lifestyle change' or 'just trying to be a bit healthier'. But thanks to the insidious nature of diet culture, our well-intended attempts at feeling better usually involve trying to control what, when, and how much we eat. We are taught that feeling better means losing weight and meeting an arbitrary aesthetic ideal. We're told that weight loss is possible for everyone. We're also taught that weight loss is uniformly a positive thing and something we should all pursue for the sake of our health. But is it as straightforward as that? There are physical, psychological, social, and behavioural consequences to dieting that no one ever talks about. Well, at least not the health and fitness mags, or the fashion mags, or the fitness influencers, or even your doctor. So, let's break it down.

This section is suitable for people with active eating disorders. There are a bunch of tools and skills contained here that will help support your eating disorder recovery

SIDE EFFECTS OF DIETS THAT NOBODY REALLY TALKS ABOUT

Food preoccupation: You know that feeling when you're on some form of diet and you can't stop scrolling through Instagram looking for recipes that contain only 'natural sugar' or are a low-carb equivalent of the food you'd actually like to eat. Our thoughts are taken over by when we can have our next meal or snack, or how many calories we're 'allowed' to eat for the rest of the day. Food preoccupation is when our headspace is filled with ideas about 'good' and 'bad' foods, rather than things we value or that bring us joy and contentment, or simply dealing with whatever shit we have going on in our lives.

Disrupts our internal cues: Dieting has been shown to disrupt the hormones that help signal hunger and fullness for up to two years after a diet stops! As well as the hormonal disruptions, ignoring or overriding your hunger can atrophy your hunger cues, making them harder to notice. [1–5]

Slowed metabolism: When I say metabolism, people often assume that I mean how quickly we burn through calories. What I really mean by metabolism, though, are all the essential functions and biochemical reactions that take place in our bodies. The net effect of eating less will obviously mean that our bodies become less efficient at these biochemical reactions and subsequently burn less energy. What is more concerning to me is that as a result of slowed biochemical reactions, our body slows down as a whole: our digestive tract becomes sluggish (causing problems like bloating and IBS-like symptoms), we may have an irregular menstrual cycle (or it may go AWOL altogether), injuries take longer to heal, and it's harder for our bodies to fight infection. So yes, our bodies burn fewer calories, but that's only a symptom of bigger problems.[6]

Disordered eating and eating disorders: Dieting is often socially sanctioned disordered eating. But because diet culture has normalized things like fasting, counting calories/macros/points, and cutting out whole food groups, we barely bat an eyelid. Long-term studies also clearly demonstrate that dieting is a risk factor for predicting the development of eating disorders. Whereas intuitive eating appears to be protective against the development of eating disorders.

Lower mood: Calorie restriction has been associated with the 'deadening of emotions'. Being on a diet can deplete serotonin production, which has an impact on our mood. More specifically, reducing our intake of carbohydrate can lead to changes in brain chemistry which can increase feelings of anxiety and food guilt. [6–7]

Poor body image: We are taught that if we're not happy with our bodies, we should change them. However, diets don't cure negative body image, and may in fact increase body preoccupation and leave us feeling worse about our bodies. Research shows that girls as young as five years old are worried about their appearance, and that 20 per cent of five-year-olds report having been on a diet![8]

Feeling addicted to food: When we remove foods from our diet, or reduce the amount of energy we're consuming, it can lead to something known as 'disinhibited' eating. This means we feel like we're out of control around food and that we will never get enough to fill us up. This is a by-product of restriction and dials way down when we are eating foods we enjoy and that are satisfying.[9]

Nutrient deficiencies: Eating less food increases the risk of missing out on key vitamins and minerals, as well as not getting enough energy from proteins, fats, and carbohydrates. Something I see quite commonly in clinic is people getting less calcium than they need because they have replaced dairy milk with non-fortified dairy alternatives (like oat or almond milk). People often choose the organic versions, thinking they are healthier, but under EU regulations, organic plant-based milks are not fortified with essential nutrients like vitamin D, calcium and iodine, making it more difficult to meet our bodies' needs.

Injuries, stress fractures, and infections: When we are in an energy deficit we might be more vulnerable to injuries, stress fractures, and infections. And they're more likely to take longer to heal and repair too, particularly if we're putting a lot of stress on our bodies through over-exercising, undernutrition, and general life stress.

Think about whether you've experienced any of these side effects; we'll take an inventory in a bit.

DO DIETS WORK?

The short answer is yes. They 'work' for a little while. But in the long term, the scientific evidence (and most people's personal experience) tells us that weight loss is incredibly difficult to achieve in the first place, and probably even harder to maintain over time. While diet culture tells us that is our own fault – that we are weak, have no willpower, and just need to try harder – the biology of dieting tells us something very different. Here are some key stats that help put this into perspective.

* If your starting BMI is 30–34.9, the annual probability of achieving a BMI of less than 24.9 is:
  - male 0.48 per cent
  - female 0.8 per cent

* If your starting BMI is 40–44.9, the annual probability of achieving a BMI of less than 24.9 is:
  - male 0.077 per cent
  - female 0.15 per cent[10]

* A large study of commercial weight-loss programmes (like Weight Watchers, Slimming World, and the like) found that 63 per cent of participants failed to lose their target of 5 per cent of body weight[11]
  - The same study also found that it cost around $155 (that's around £125) to lose 1 kilogram on Weight Watchers.
  - And $424 (£340) per kilogram on Jenny Craig.

* Another large study which pooled together 29 smaller studies found that after losing weight, people tended to gain back up to 50 per cent of the weight they had lost after two years and up to 80 per cent after 5 years.[12]

Those are some pretty dismal stats, and the idea that diets don't work long-term is not controversial in nutritional science: it's been a well-established phenomenon since the 1940s. But despite all we know about the ineffectiveness of dieting, the global diet and fitness industry was worth £151 billion in 2018, highlighting just how influential and pervasive diet culture is.[13] Diet companies make bank on this, except instead of owning up to their shitty products and shady practices, they have the audacity to blame us when we can't maintain weight loss in the long term, and then try and sell us another diet! This is how we get trapped in the diet cycle – a never-ending merry-go-round of weight-loss attempts, characterized by spectacularly falling off the wagon, only to convince ourselves that it was our own fault, and hopping straight back on. Let's take a closer look at how this works.

The diet cycle

1 **Desire to be thin:** We receive messages from diet culture that our lives would be better, and we would be healthier, *if* we lost weight. So, we embark on a new diet, healthy lifestyle, or wellness regimen.

2 **Restrictive diet:** We start cutting out foods, food groups, or simply start counting things. You might ditch gluten, dairy, refined sugar, and anything 'processed'. You might also double down on your HIIT classes or gym sessions.

3 **Diet mentality:** This is where food preoccupation sets in and you become hyper-vigilant about your food choices. You might start obsessively checking food labels, or tracking everything in a fitness app, or checking to make sure there's something 'clean' on the menu before you go out to dinner. You might also notice yourself body-checking in the mirror more often.

4 Weight loss: You might initially notice some changes in your body – this will likely be a combination of fat, glycogen from your muscles (aka 'water weight'), and protein from muscle breakdown. This might give you a little temporary bump in encouragement.

5 Hunger and cravings set in: Our body doesn't understand that there isn't a food shortage, and adapts by making changes to our brain chemistry, resulting in increased and intensified hunger signals and cravings. It's thought that for every kilogram lost, appetite increases by around an additional 100 kcal per day compared to before weight loss.[13]

6 Blowout: The food preoccupation, the unsustainable exercise regimen, and the increased hunger all culminate after a long, stressful day, where you say *'fuck it'* and eat what subjectively feels like a lot of food. It may also feel out of control or 'disinhibited'.

7 Guilt and anxiety: Because of the chemical changes in the brain from restricting, and because of the shame diet culture has baked into us, we inevitably feel terrible for breaking the diet. We might also find that once we've fallen off the wagon, we (understandably) don't want to get back on. The blowout may last days, weeks, or even longer. As we'll discuss, even the threat of restriction can cause this backlash of blowout eating.

8 Weight gain: Our bodies return to the weight they were at prior to the diet – they may even add on a 'cushion' in preparation for another enforced period of restriction in the future. We're back to the top of the cycle again. And because we've internalized the idea that weight gain is bad, we might be tempted to restart the cycle again and go on another diet.

Does this cycle feel familiar to you? Over what time period do you typically experience this cycle – years, months, weeks, or even within a single day? Can you identify where you are on the cycle right now? How many times have you been round this cycle?

HOW TO BREAK UP WITH DIET CULTURE

Breaking up with the allure and promise of dieting is tough; even people who have been practising intuitive eating for many years sometimes feel diet mentality thoughts creep in. It's hardly surprising when we stop and notice how deeply fat-phobic society is, and the incessant nature of diet culture. So it's important that we give ourselves a break when we notice the draw back to dieting.

The next section will walk you through the following steps to help you ditch the diet mentality:

1 The cost of restriction Recognize that diets are not harmless – understand the side effects that diets can have.

2 Your relationship with food Understand how diets have personally impacted you and your relationship with food; how they've taken a toll on your mental and physical health.

3 Dieting expectations vs reality Push back on diet culture and get mad as hell about the lies it has sold you.

4 Social media diet culture detox Unhook yourself from diet tools by holding a Fitbit funeral.

5 Be kind to yourself – head back to your toolkit if you've been through the steps above, or check out the self-compassion practice in Chapter 5.

If you feel that pull back towards dieting at any point, then return to this section of the book whenever you need to.

THE COST OF RESTRICTION

For some people diets 'work'. I hear all the time from people who tell me they've maintained a significant weight loss for a sustained period. All they did was cut out all sugar and carbs, only eat 'clean' food, quit their job in finance to become a full-time fitness instructor, and never sit down for more than fifteen minutes at a time. I'm only half joking here; people go to enormous lengths and make huge sacrifices just to weigh a little bit less. This is a completely personal decision, and I'm not here to judge anyone's choices, but I am here if you feel like the cost of trying to control and manipulate your body is becoming too high, and you want a way out. Let's take stock of what dieting has cost you personally. That way you can make an informed decision about whether or not it's still working for you.

 Check the boxes next to the side effects of dieting you have experienced. There's space at the bottom of each column to add your own.

Psychological	Physical	Social	Relationships	Behavioural
☐ Food preoccupation	☐ Malnutrition/ nutrient deficiency	☐ Missing out on important social events/occasions	☐ Caused problems in my romantic relationship(s)	☐ Binge eating/feeling out of control around food
☐ Eating disorder/ disordered eating	☐ Weight cycling (yo-yo dieting)	☐ Being unable to connect with loved ones due to worrying about food	☐ Caused difficulties with my friendships	☐ Going to the gym and sacrificing rest/sleep
☐ Low mood (anxiety/ depression)	☐ Increased cortisol (stress hormone)	☐ Social isolation (not seeing friends/loved ones because you're at the gym/don't want to eat out at a restaurant, etc)	☐ Challenged my relationship with my kids	☐ Obsessively tracking exercise, calories, macros or points
☐ Body-bashing and poor body image	☐ Recurring infections	☐ Not able to join in with holiday foods (Christmas, Easter, Thanksgiving, Hanukah, etc)	☐ Taken a toll on my relationship with siblings/parents	☐ Weighing food
☐ Feeling addicted to food	☐ Taking a long time to recover between workouts		☐ Affected my relationship with colleagues	☐ Weighing yourself regularly (and it dictating how you feel)
	☐ Low energy and fatigue			
	☐ Low bone density/ stress fractures			
	☐ Feeling dizzy/faint from low blood sugar/hunger			

> Has dieting affected you in ways that surprised you or you hadn't realized before?

YOUR RELATIONSHIP WITH FOOD

Let's take a closer look at how our relationship with food got so complicated in the first place, and where dieting first made its appearance. In your journal, I'd like you to write about – or draw a timeline to illustrate – how your relationship with food has evolved over time. Start with childhood, and work your way forward through that very first diet, all the way up until now. Use the following prompts to help you.

* Growing up, what was your parent(s)'/caregiver(s)' relationship to food like? (Repeat this for any relatives that had a significant presence while you were growing up.)

- Did they diet or otherwise manipulate their food intake?

- Did they label certain foods as good/bad?

- Did they use food as reward or punishment?

- What were their attitudes to different body sizes?

- Did they revere thinner bodies while disparaging bigger bodies?

- How did they talk about and treat their own body?

- What was their relationship with movement and exercise?

- Did you have enough food to eat as a child or did you live with food insecurity?

> Please note, the intention behind these questions is not to shame or judge the people who raised us; it's simply an opportunity to reflect on the genesis of some of these difficulties. Keep in mind that our relatives are swimming through the same soup of diet culture as we are.

HOW TO JUST EAT IT

* When did you first notice your body wasn't 'good enough'?

* What do you think contributed to these feelings?

* Did family and friends comment on your eating behaviours or body size (positively or negatively)?

* When did you first attempt to manipulate your body through diet and exercise?

  - List the various diets you've attempted over the years – including the 'healthy lifestyles', the 'wellness' diets and other diets in disguise.

  - Did they coincide with any important life events or periods of difficulty?

  - How has dieting been a way of helping you cope or survive difficult times?

  - What has the financial cost of dieting been? Can you tally up the amount you have spent on diet programmes, gym memberships, wellness foods and other products diet culture tells us we 'need?'

* How might dieting have been a coping mechanism for you? For instance, a way to cope when things felt overwhelming? Did dieting provide a sense of safety or community? Perhaps it offered a reprieve from experiencing stigma? Perhaps it was a means of seeking out acceptance?

+ How did these formative experiences affect how you feel about food and your body now?

+ List the ways dieting has made your life better/easier, and how it might have made things more difficult/challenging.

Take your time – It can be difficult to reflect on these questions, so take it slow; and if it becomes too much, step away until you're in a better place to think about these things. Also, if this is touching on trauma then consider reaching out for support – I know professional support is an enormous privilege, so if it's not accessible to you, consider support available to you through friends and communities. Do what you need to do to look after yourself.

YOUR BRAIN ON EXTERNAL RULES VS YOUR BRAIN AS AN INTUITIVE EATER

When we are dieting or caught up in disordered eating patterns, food and exercise seem to take over our brain, leaving little space for more fulfilling or enjoyable activities. Some clients have told me that 80–90 per cent of their headspace is occupied by thoughts about food, nutrition, and body hatred. Finding peace with food and our bodies can free up space for us to focus on the things that really matter to us.

Using the template below, draw out how much space you feel is currently taken up by thoughts of food, exercise, dieting, weight and body concerns while on a diet or subscribing to diet culture. Remember, 'diet' here is shorthand for all of the rules and restriction we've internalized, even if we're not on an official diet. It can be helpful to write out the specific thoughts or concerns, showing how much space they occupy.

....

On a diet

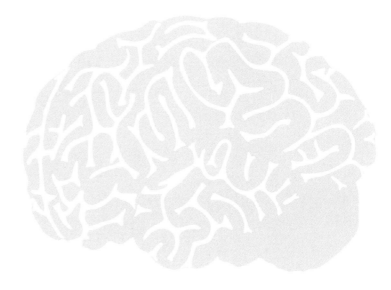

* What proportion of your headspace is dedicated to thinking about food, diet, exercise, etc?

* Were you surprised at how much brain space is taken up worrying about food and exercise?

* What else would you like to fill your brain up with? Consider your hobbies and interests, or refer back to your list of values for inspiration.

On this next template, draw or write out what other passions and activities you'd like to fill your brain with if you had more semblance of balance in your life. Food and movement can feature here, but the key is to think about the kind of balance that you want to achieve between those and your other interests.

As an intuitive eater

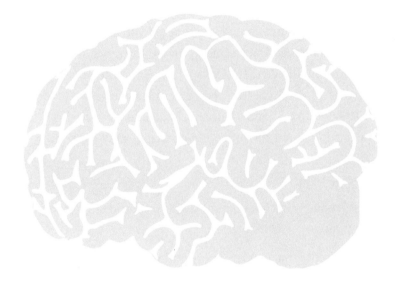

* Is there anything you've listed that you could start taking steps towards right now, in your right now body?

* We often get caught up in the idea that we'll do a thing when we weigh X. Is there anything we might have missed out on while waiting for the scales to give us the green light?

* What is really stopping us from doing that thing right now?

DIETING EXPECTATIONS VS REALITY

As you go through the process of intuitive eating, it's pretty normal to second-guess whether or not you should try one last diet. As you learn to make peace with food, and understand that all foods are equal, you might feel like you're regularly eating past comfortable fullness or are out of control, and maybe you're worried about gaining weight. It becomes tempting to think that a diet will be the solution: maybe if you just lose X number of pounds you'll be happy with your body and THEN you can give this intuitive eating thing a go. But here's the thing: dieting doesn't fix poor body image. It doesn't heal your relationship with food. It's helpful to take some time to reflect on what you expected from dieting and where it got you in the past.

 In your journal, draw a line to divide the page in two and add the headings EXPECTATIONS vs REALITY. Note down your own experiences in each column. For example, 'I'll be very good and follow the diet to a T' and 'I felt restricted and overate "bad" foods'. Having a think about the following questions may help you.

* Does dieting make you obsessive about food and body image?

* Do you put your life on hold waiting for the day you reach that elusive clothes size?

* Does dieting make you cranky and miserable?

* Do you stop seeing your friends for dinner or drinks?

* Does it impact your relationship with your partner, or ability to be present in other areas of life (career, kids, education, creative pursuits)?

* What are the issues and problems I'm facing right now in my life?

* If I'm being honest, will these problems really be fixed by losing weight, or is there something else behind this desire?

SOCIAL MEDIA DIET CULTURE DETOX

We all use social media differently, and the ways it can influence how we feel about food and our bodies is complicated. However, some research has indicated that social media can negatively impact our relationship with food and our bodies, and is related to disordered eating. For instance, studies have noted that:

* 1 in 5 UK adults said that images on social media caused them to worry about their body image.

* 87 per cent of women and 65 per cent of men compare their bodies to images they consume on social and traditional media.[14]

* Viewing #fitspo (from 'fit-inspiration') on Instagram leads to self-compassion going down, compared to viewing self-compassion quotes, which helped buffer the impact of #fitspo.[15]

* As many as 90 per cent of women who participated in 'healthy eating' communities on Instagram had symptoms that aligned with orthorexia nervosa (an unhealthy obsession with healthy eating).[16]

* Looking at #BoPo (that's short for 'body positive') accounts on Instagram helped improve mood, body satisfaction, and body appreciation, relative to thin-ideal and appearance-neutral posts. However, viewing both the BoPo and thin-ideal images increased self-objectification, leading the authors of this study to wonder if having such an intense focus on bodies was helpful. In other words, focusing on bodies can lead us to forget that our physical shells are not as important as our characteristics, talents, and skills.[17]

* Although most body image research is done on women, research has shown that men who spend a lot of time looking at #fitspo are more likely to work out for aesthetic

as opposed to being motivated by improving their health. Looking at more #fitspo was associated with less body satisfaction overall.[18]

Given the pervasiveness of diet culture in social media, and its subsequent influence over how we feel about food and our bodies – doesn't it make sense to sort that shit out? Typically, in one of the first few sessions I have with a client, I'll ask them to whip out their phones so we can talk through who they're following on Instagram and why. I'll ask, 'Does this person make you feel good about yourself?' Even if you've been through and had a social media clear-out in the past, it can be helpful to check back in with a fresh pair of eyes and get really real with yourself. Here are some of the things my team at LCIE look out for.

Red flags

* Transformation pics

* Diet products – shapewear, supplements, activewear that's not size inclusive

* Lack of diversity

* Pictures carefully posed to look thin (or doubled over to show off 'belly rolls')

* Meal prep

* Comparisons of portions, calories, macros

* Lack of white, beige, brown foods – any potatoes?

* Food groups missing from pics

* 'Perfect' meals – no sign of canned, frozen, ready-prepared food

* Inconsistent messages – weight loss one day; how to handle emotional eating the next

* Treating eating over an occasion (Christmas, weddings) as a problem, and suggesting ways to cope with it

* Promotion of some foods and snacks as 'healthy', putting them on a pedestal over other foods

* Adapting fun foods into 'healthy' versions

Questions to ask yourself

* Who do they follow? Is there diversity and a range of interests?

* If you cover up the pictures, how do the words make you feel?

* If you cover up the words, how do the pictures make you feel?

* Is it making you feel good about the food you're seeing, or bad about the food you're eating?

* Are they promoting their own diets and exercise schedules with the suggestion that you can look like they do?

So pour yourself something to drink and reflect on the above points while you're sipping and scrolling. Don't be afraid to be liberal with that unfollow button, and if you can't unfollow for political reasons (friends, family, mutual friends, colleagues or clients), you can always mute posts. In the Resources section you'll find a list of my favourite body liberation activists, researchers, and anti-diet professionals to follow instead – clients have told me that following these folks really helps facilitate the intuitive eating process and makes them feel less crappy about themselves when they're online.

Don't forget that little caveat though, that focusing all your attention on bodies may not be that helpful, so as you're reflecting on your feed, notice if it's skewed more towards #fitspo, hot celebs, fashion models, yummy mummies, and other beautiful people. Or does it reflect all of your interests and hobbies? Is there stuff there that engages your brain, along with the cute dog pics and hilarious memes? Is your social media a reflection of you as a whole?

How do you feel now that you've cleared out your social media and had a diet culture detox? Does your social media feel like a place where you actually want to hang out now? Do you feel inspired and uplifted by social media (as opposed to feeling bad about yourself)? Keep reflecting on who you are following and why and periodically give your socials a spring clean.

Softening Our Gaze and Zooming Out

Nadia Craddock, PhD
Body image researcher
and co-host of
Appearance Matters
and The Body Protest
podcasts.
@nadia.craddock

It is very common to be hypercritical of our own appearance, particularly when we come face to face with it – for example, looking in the mirror or seeing photos of ourselves on social media. When we are struggling with our relationship with our body, we tend to zoom in on perceived imperfections, rather than seeing the bigger picture of our bodies and our whole selves. It is all too easy to get caught in a trap of constantly scrutinizing, monitoring and comparing our appearance. If you are in this head space, remember:

1 you are not alone, and

2 you don't have to stay there; it's possible to change how you think, feel, and relate to your body.

Objectification Theory

Objectification Theory is a feminist theory on body image, first put forward by Barbara Fredrickson and Tomi-Ann Roberts in 1997, that offers an explanation as to why we are so critical of our appearance and how this can affect our body image, mood, and our relationship to food. The theory argues that girls and women are 'acculturated to internalize an observer's perspective as a primary view of their physical selves' – that is, girls and women are socially conditioned to be constantly aware of their appearance and how they are viewed by others. This observer's perspective is often spoken about in relation to the 'male gaze' (a term coined by film critic Laura Mulvey), the way in which men often sexually objectify women's bodies in society, reducing women to their bodies. Old-school advertising is a classic example of this, where women are positioned and posed as passive objects of (heteronormative) male desire. Catcalling in the street ('nice tits, love') is another form of sexual objectification.

In response to both consuming and experiencing sexual objectification, girls and women may internalize the belief that their worth is contingent upon how closely their body approximates society's appearance ideals. In turn, they are more likely to engage in habitual patterns of self-scrutiny and self-monitoring ('self-surveillance') of their appearance, which can heighten appearance anxiety and body shame (a sense of failure for not meeting general or specific appearance standards), as well as disordered eating and depressed mood.

There are a lot of references to 'girls and women' in the explanation above, reflecting the original outline of the theory. However, while most of the evidence supporting the theory has focused on cisgender women, more recent research finds support for the theory among people with different gender identities, including transgender men and women, and gay cisgender men.[19, 20, 21]

Objectification and social media

The relationship between objectification and body image is particularly pertinent in the context of social media. In addition to the likelihood of consuming objectifying images, we are also turning the camera on ourselves and sharing our own image for others to look at. This may exacerbate our external view of ourselves and our preoccupation with how others see us. Viewers' likes and comments also serve as a tangible marker of how our image is being perceived, which may heighten appearance anxiety and preoccupation with our (online) image. The use of apps and filters may encourage greater scrutiny of our appearance as we (subconsciously) compare our unedited and edited images. Engaging in self-objectification and/or appearance comparisons are two important mechanisms explaining research that finds positive correlations between social media use, body image, mood, and disordered eating.[22, 23] When you feel yourself falling into the hypercritical head space, try one of these exercises.

Zooming out

✖ Your body is more than your appearance. Your body may allow you to do a range of things that give you pleasure and fulfilment or simply allow you to be and carry out day-to-day tasks. Our bodies are all different: yours may allow you to move, participate in sports, carry the shopping, paint a picture, play a musical instrument, hug someone you love, read a book, listen to music, watch the sunset. Try to zoom out and think about all the things your body allows you to do.

✖ Your appearance is not your worth. You are a multi-faceted human with talents, skills, values, thoughts, emotions, and ideas. You are not an oil painting. Try to **zoom out and think about your whole self.**

✖ If you find yourself stressing over how you look in a photo on social media, try to **zoom out and think of positives captured in the photo.** Who are you with? Where are you? What did you do that day?

Softening your gaze

✖ When you catch yourself engaging in unkind, critical thoughts about your body, **soften your gaze** and your inner dialogue.

✖ If find yourself pinching or prodding parts of your body you don't like, **soften your touch** and perhaps stroke or pat that body part, reminding yourself you are just right.

FITBIT FUNERAL

Someone once sent me a DM saying they held a Fitbit funeral as part of their eating disorder recovery treatment – I thought it was a perfect name for ditching the tools of dieting because it sums up the fact that there is a grieving and mourning process that takes place when we move away from diet culture. So, thank you to the person who shared this with me – wish I knew your name so I could credit you!

External monitors distract us from and make it difficult to recognize internal cues – they foster distrust in our body. So, I want you to consider stepping away from the Fitbit. I know that dieting tools often feel like a safety net for people – I'm talking calorie-counting apps, step counters, activity trackers, diet books, rigid meal plans, workout programmes, and the rest. They give us a sense of security in an otherwise unpredictable world, so it makes total sense if you're not ready to ditch all of these at once. Let's take it step by step.

1   Write out all of your diet tools in order of most scary to give up (at the top) to least scary to give up.

2   Remind yourself why you don't need them.

   ∗ In a sample of around 100 people with an eating disorder, 75 per cent were using MyFitnessPal to track calories; of those, 73 per cent agreed that MFP was a contributing factor to eating disorder symptoms and behaviours.[24]

   ∗ Research on calorie-tracking apps suggests that the feedback on MyFitnessPal may lead to a restrictive, unbalanced diet.[25]

   ∗ Apps and digital tools can lead to 'techorexia' – a term coined to describe compulsive behaviour normalized by the popularization of health-monitoring tech.[26]

＊ Fitness and calorie trackers are associated with eating disorder symptoms, and negative body image, even in people who do not have diagnosed eating disorders.[27]

3   Decide which tool you're ready to experiment with letting go of. If you're feeling confident then pick something higher up your list; if not, pick something a bit lower down.

4   How long are you going to commit to letting go of this tool? It may be indefinitely, it may just be a few hours, or to go for one run without your fitness tracker – decide what you feel comfortable with.

5   Check in with your intuitive eating toolkit. Which tools and skills can you draw on to make it easier for yourself? What self-care practices might help make the transition easier?

6   Afterwards, check in with yourself – how did it go? What went well? What did you learn from this experience that might help you next time?

7   Rinse and repeat: keep practising this activity until you've ditched all the diet tools.

What was scariest about stepping away from these tools?
Was there anything liberating or freeing about this experience?
What might help you ditch those last few tools?

DIET CULTURE BULLSHIT BINGO

Diet culture is everywhere: in magazines, on social media, in advertising, movies, TV shows, on the news, in our doctor's surgery, on our food packaging. Once you start to notice it, it can feel overwhelming: a never-ending barrage of messages with the subtext that you'd be a better human if you lost weight. I get how crushing this can be, and I promise you'll reach a point where you feel a lot more resilient to it and can laugh or shrug it off. In the meantime, you can call out the diet culture bullshit with this bingo template. Feel free to add any more examples that you come across to the blank squares.

'Earning' food with exercise	Cheat day/ meal	It's not a diet, it's a lifestyle!	80/20 rule	Eat everything in moderation	Sugar is as addictive as heroin
Lose weight the healthy way!	All natural	'Burning off' food		Are you hungry or just thirsty?	Gym mirror selfies
Shred, burn, and blast	Before/after weight-loss pictures	Appetite suppressant	Fat jokes/ stereotypes	Low calorie	'Sculpt' a body part (butt, thighs, etc)
Guilt-free	Detox		If it fits your macros	'Light' versions of foods	
Portion control		Photos of headless fatties	Cauliflower pizza	'Thinspiration'	Meal prep photos that don't contain any carbs
	Lack of body diversity (thin, white, able-bodied only)	No refined sugar	Cleanse		

How long did it take you to get a full house or thereabouts?
Had you noticed the prevalence of diet culture messaging before now?

+ How does changing up your social media impact how you feel about food and your body?

+ Has the cost of dieting been higher than you realized?

+ What fairy lights have turned on for you?

+ Are there any tools from this section that you can add to your toolkit? Go back to Chapter 1 and write them in.

In your journal, make a note of the answers to the following questions

Listen to the corresponding podcast episode Don't Salt My Game – How to Just Eat It: Chapter 3

CHAPTER 3

GETTING TO KNOW HUNGER

For people with eating disorders, getting familiar with the signals for hunger is critical, as is learning that hunger isn't a bad thing. However, you might not reliably be able to recognise and follow hunger signals because eating disorders have a tendency to undermine them. Talk to your treatment team about how you can begin to recognize hunger signals while following a meal plan.

Add to this list

OK, time to get down to business. In this section we're going to explore how we can reconnect to physical sensations of hunger in our bodies. Let me start by asking you a question: have you ever done any of the following as a way of trying to pacify or soothe feelings of hunger?

- ☐ Drink a glass of water
- ☐ Smoke a cigarette
- ☐ Have a cup of tea or coffee
- ☐ Pour yourself some wine
- ☐ Have a Diet Coke
- ☐ Chew gum
- ☐ Go to bed early
- ☐ Straight up ignore it
- ☐ ....
- ☐ ....
- ☐ ....

My guess is that you probably checked at least one of the boxes above. And this isn't unusual. We are conditioned to believe that we can't trust our bodies to guide our eating. Ever been told 'you're not hungry, you're just thirsty'? *Exactly!* We trust apps on our phones more than we trust our body's innate wisdom. And it makes sense, right? That strong connection to our eating instinct can become worn down through decades of societal programming for what, when, and how we 'should' eat, and what our bodies 'should' look like. The good news is that instinct is still there; even people who have had severe eating disorders can reconnect with their intuitive eater given the right support.[1]

Fundamentally, hunger is a normal biological function; it helps us gauge when our body is running low on fuel and we need to top up the tank. However, through dieting and wellness culture, we learn to override our hunger, or we eat less than we really need to feel satisfied. There are a couple of side effects to this:

1 We are constantly thinking about food! We feel completely obsessed with it. It's not until we feel regularly satisfied that our brain stops thinking about it. This is known as food preoccupation.

2 We feel out of control around food. We might regularly eat past the point of comfortable fullness – not because we are weak-willed or 'greedy', but because we have been underfeeding ourselves, causing our biology to fight back and ask to be fed! We end up swinging from being way past gentle hunger to uncomfortably full, rather than from gentle hunger to comfortable fullness.

Hunger is one of the most basic instincts we have as humans, yet we systematically override or ignore hunger sensations. We wouldn't try and hold back peeing, pooping, coughing, or sneezing, yet we try and pretend hunger isn't happening to us unless we are so ravenous that we're about to pass out.

INTEROCEPTIVE AWARENESS

You've probably heard people say things like 'listen to your body'; what they don't tell you is *how* or *why*. This concept sounds a bit nebulous and unscientific, but in the realm of nutritional science we have a name for listening to your body: *interoceptive awareness*.[2] Interoceptive awareness is a way of saying that we have a strong mind–body connection – information is gathered from our body and processed in our minds, whether this is recognizing emotions that originate in the body, perceiving our heart rate, a full bladder, feeling sleepy, or the need to sneeze. We can also perceive food-related information being sent by the body – hunger, fullness, cravings, satiation, satisfaction, thirst, and energy levels. In other words, the signals for eating intuitively are all there, and studies have shown that intuitive eaters tend to have higher interoceptive awareness.[3] Problem is, these signals can become dampened and desensitized through external cues. Interoceptive awareness is an *inside job*, so it makes sense that when we look outside of ourselves for rules about what, when, and how much to eat, we lose touch with these cues.

Our body image can also mess with our interoceptive sensitivity. Self-objectification refers to the idea that, in a culture that objectifies the female body, women and increasingly folks of other genders are vigilantly aware of their outer body appearance; they may be left with fewer perceptual resources available for recognizing and responding to internal cues like hunger and satiety, heartbeat, and perceived blood glucose levels. There's also an argument that self-objectification encourages folks to go on diets to try and control their weight, and therefore appearance, which also desensitizes them to physiological cues. If you're constantly thinking about your outward appearance, you've got less internal awareness of what's going on inside your body.

Not getting enough rest and good-quality sleep can also perturb our interoceptive awareness, as can having certain mental health conditions, including eating disorders – in fact, having low interoceptive awareness is considered to be a hallmark of an eating disorder. Tribole and Resch conceptualize that intuitive eating helps improve interoceptive awareness in two ways: **1** by removing barriers to interoceptive awareness, and **2** by directly cultivating stronger interoceptive awareness.[4*]

Removing barriers to interoceptive awareness	Cultivating stronger interoceptive awareness
Reject the diet mentality – stop all forms of dieting, behaviourally and mentally	Honour your hunger – eat when you are biologically hungry
Make peace with food – no food is forbidden; eat all the foods you desire, based on attunement to hunger and fullness cues	Respect your fullness – stop eating when comfortably full, not too little and not too much
Challenge the food police – question your food rules, which may originate in personal, family, and cultural beliefs	Discover the satisfaction factor – aim for satisfaction when eating meals and snacks
Cope with your emotions with kindness – use a variety of skills to deal with difficult feelings and emotions	Exercise, feel the difference – discover enjoyable ways to move the body
Respect your body – your body deserves to be treated with dignity and respect, regardless of shape or size	
Honour your health with gentle nutrition – select foods that taste good and make you feel well	

* Some neurodivergent folks may have difficulty sensing some cues like hunger and thirst so may need additional structure, such as a regular meal and snack schedule. There is no judgement or shame here for relying on external cues for self-care.

The good news is that interoceptive awareness can be rediscovered, even if it's buried way down deep under loads of dieting rules.

Perceive your own heart rate

If you have a smart watch or fitness tracker (yes, I know I told you to get rid, but just for experiment's sake) you can objectively measure your own heart rate, while subjectively guesstimating by tuning into the perception of your heart beating.

 Sit in a quiet room where you won't be disturbed. Allow yourself a few minutes for your heart rate to come to rest if you've been up and about – two to three minutes will be enough. Start a timer for one minute, then set your watch to start counting, but try not to look at it. Meanwhile notice where you can feel your heartbeat – perhaps you can feel a gentle beating in your chest, or a light pulsing in your neck or fingers. Count the beats or pulses for the full minute. Afterwards you can compare the numbers of the objective heart rate monitor to your perceived heart rate.

* Measured heart rate _____ bpm

* Subjective heart rate _____ bpm

* If you were able to detect your own heartbeat, where did you feel it most strongly?

* How closely did the numbers align?

* How did you find this activity? Was it simple and intriguing, or challenging and frustrating?

* Was there anything that got in the way of tuning in? (e.g. distractions, critical self-talk)

* Was there anything else interesting that you observed?

Don't worry if you weren't able to perceive your heart rate accurately (or at all). If you've been following external rules for a long time, it can take a while to get back to internal signals. Try to cultivate a little compassion for yourself; the following activities will help you get more in touch with physical sensations. You might want to come back to this activity periodically to see if that connection feels like it's getting stronger.

CONCEPTUALIZING HUNGER

We can imagine hunger and fullness like a fuel gauge in your car that goes from zero to ten. Zero is so empty, you're basically running on fumes, and you might feel sick, dizzy, or faint. At 10 the tank is spilling over. It's so uncomfortably full that again you might feel sick. Five is neutral, content and comfortable, neither empty nor full – this is often how we feel between meals or snacks, when we're not really thinking about food. The following diagram can be used to help us understand how this relates to our bodies; here I've filled it out to show how clients tend to experience sensations of hunger and fullness in their bodies, but there's a blank template in the appendix for you to fill in your own.

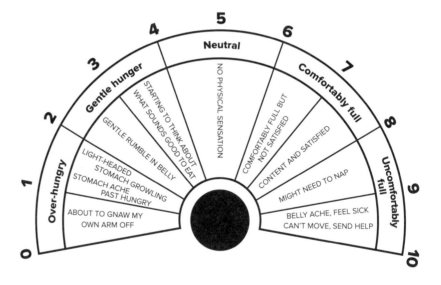

* Think about a time when you were really low on fuel (overhungry) – down below a 2 on the hunger wheel. How did it feel? What physical sensations did you notice?

* What was your subsequent experience with food? Did you eat calmly and mindfully, paying attention to the textures or

flavours? Or did you hoover it down while standing over the kitchen sink?

✱ How did it feel after you'd eaten? What were the physical sensations? What were your thoughts and feelings?

✱ How do you think the experience might have differed if you'd eaten when you were gently hungry (a 3 or 4)?

Typically, when we let ourselves get *over*-hungry (intentionally or otherwise), eating feels chaotic and out of control. It reinforces the idea that we can't be trusted around food, causing us to further control and restrict what we eat. But what we have a harder time recognizing is that overshooting our fullness levels is a normal response to restriction and deprivation; it's our body's way of trying to keep us safe. Still, many of us feel that we shouldn't or aren't 'allowed' to eat until we experience a level of hunger that makes us feel physically ill. It might help to keep in mind that hunger isn't meant to be pathological – it shouldn't be associated with pain and suffering. Mild discomfort, sure. But it shouldn't hurt or make you miserable; if it does, that's a pretty solid sign that you're over-hungry!

RECONNECTING WITH HUNGER

Adapted from Tribole &
Resch, intuitiveeating.org

It might surprise you to learn that hunger isn't *just* in our stomach. Yet most people wait until there's a deeply uncomfortable emptiness or growling in the pit of their stomach before eating – this is *over-hunger*. In order to start re-establishing a connection with our body, we need to learn to recognize all the subtle cues our body is sending us. My favourite way to do this is with a hunger body scan.

Hunger body scan

Record the following script on your phone and use it to get in touch with the sensations your body is signalling to indicate you're hungry!

Get yourself nice and comfortable, sitting with your feet planted on the floor and a tall, straight spine. If it feels OK, gently close your eyes, otherwise gaze down at a spot on the floor in front of you . . .

Begin by taking a few deep breaths, in through your nose and out through your mouth . . . In through your nose and out through your mouth. And once more, breathing in through your nose and out through your mouth . . .

Let's start getting in touch with your physical body . . .

In your head, scan your body, starting from your head and moving down towards your toes . . .

How would you describe the physical sensations in your body in this moment? . . . Are they pleasant? . . . Unpleasant? . . . Or neutral? . . . There's no right or wrong answer, you're just checking in with yourself. Just notice the description that best describes how you physically feel, right now . . .

Now we're going to look at some key areas where hunger can show up in the body, starting with the more subtle and nuanced signs of hunger . . .

Bring your attention to your mood . . .

Sometimes biological hunger is experienced with a shift in mood. You may feel irritable or cranky . . . Notice your mood right now in this moment . . . Do you feel a little snappy? . . . Do you feel a little low? . . .

If so, these may be signs that you're beginning to experience hunger. Just take notice, without judgement . . .

Shift your attention to your overall energy level . . . Sometimes biological hunger is experienced by a dip in energy, characterized by fatigue, or even sleepiness . . . Do you feel sluggish and tired and it has nothing to do with a bad night's sleep? . . .

Again, just notice if you experience these initial signs of hunger by a shift in your energy . . .

Now I'd like you to shift your attention to the more easily detectable hunger signals, starting with your head, so just bring your awareness to your head . . .

Sometimes biological hunger is experienced as a physical sensation in your head, so just notice any physical sensations in your head right now . . . How would you describe the way it feels to you? . . .

Is there a slight ache? . . . Are you light-headed, or does it feel like you're zoning out? . . . Maybe you feel a little dizzy, or even a bit faint? . . . Are you having any difficulty concentrating? . . . Whatever the sensation, just notice it . . .

If you're experiencing any of these sensations, it's possible that you're feeling a degree of hunger . . .

Just notice it without judgement . . .

Now, move your attention to your stomach . . .

What would best describe the physical sensation in your stomach right now? . . . Would you describe it as a gentle rumbling or gurgling? . . . Or maybe it feels empty? . . . Or perhaps there's an uncomfortable pain, a stomach ache . . .

Are there any hunger pangs or a gnawing feeling in your belly? . . . Or does your stomach feel comfortable or neutral? . . .

What is the physical sensation in your stomach? Be aware that any of these sensations may be signalling hunger . . .

Perhaps you're experiencing other physical sensations that might be indicating you're hungry . . . Maybe you feel weak . . . Or maybe you feel kinda shaky and like you have low blood sugar, another physical symptom of hunger indicating you need to eat . . .

Now I'd like you to run another scan of all of these elements, starting with your mood . . .

Now your energy level . . .

Now the physical sensations, in your head and your stomach and anywhere else you might be experiencing them . . .

Consider all of these elements together, and with that overall consideration, I'd like you to rate your hunger level on a hunger/ fullness scale from 0 to 10 . . . 10 is so full you feel sick, it's painful . . . 0 is painfully empty. And 5 is completely neutral; neither empty nor full. So how would you rate your hunger right now? . . .

Keep in mind, whatever number you rate, there's no right or wrong. It's just a process to help you get in touch, and the more you get familiar with the sensations, the easier it will become to tell when you're hungry . . .

Take a few deep breaths in through your nose and out through your mouth. In through your nose and out through your mouth. And once more, in through your nose and out through your mouth. Open your eyes, and bring your attention back to the room.

> Reflect on the hunger body scan you just did — what are your immediate thoughts? Were you surprised to notice the other ways that hunger can show up in your body besides your stomach? Do you experience any of these more nuanced hunger signals?

Don't worry if you don't notice any other signs of hunger just yet. Getting back in touch with these signals is a process and takes practice. Which is exactly what we're going to do.

Hunger body scan practice

Sometimes the signs and signals around hunger don't become apparent until we no longer feel them. Ever had an awful headache, only for it to go away almost immediately after you've eaten? That's what I mean! For this practice, we're going to look at the physical sensations we experience before and after we've eaten a snack and then compare and contrast them using the table below.

Step 1: When you know you're feeling hungry (but not so hungry you feel unwell), play the body scan meditation and circle the sensations you're experiencing from the list below, or add your own. You might only know you're hungry because a significant amount of time has passed since your last meal or snack. Try and do this, if you can, at a time when you are relatively rested, calm, and have slept well. This will help you tease out what is a hunger signal versus feeling off-kilter for some other reason.

Mood	Energy	Head	Stomach	Body
irritable	fatigued	achy	gurgling	salivating
cranky	sleepy	dizzy	gentle rumbling	weak
hangry	sluggish	light-headed	empty	low blood sugar
snappy	blah	distracted	stomach ache	anxiety
low	lethargic	unfocused	hunger pangs	
	listless	poor concentration	gnawing	

Step 2: Now have a meal or snack, then wait 15–20 minutes and repeat the body scan meditation. Using a different colour pen, circle the sensations that are still present after eating.

> Can you begin to notice your own sensations of hunger? You may experience one sensation really strongly, and some others more subtly, or maybe they're all a bit subtle. Don't worry if it's not all super clear immediately. Keep practising the body scan and use this before and after technique as many times as you need to. Remember, there are no hard and fasts, it's just a process to get in touch and figure out what's going on for you.

The hunger and satisfaction guide

Another tool we can use to get in touch with hunger is the hunger and satisfaction guide. This wheel allows us to visualize the fuel gauge metaphor we used earlier. *In the appendix, there is a full-size version of this guide which you can cut out and use for this section. See page 311 for details.*

Use the word bank next to the wheel to fill in the spokes of the wheel. If you find it difficult to tell the difference between, say, a 3 and a 4, don't worry too much about it. Use the labels in the outer part of the wheel to guide eating (a 2–4 means you're hungry and it's time to eat something). We don't need to overthink it! Also, if you find the numbers unhelpful or you notice yourself trying to follow them 'perfectly', then that's another indication you might want to step back and focus on the outer part of the wheel.

What if I'm struggling to recognize my hunger?

It's very unlikely that you don't experience *any* signals for hunger – but they might be dulled and diluted, meaning we have to pay really close attention to recognize them. Fortunately, we can recalibrate our signals to give them a boost so they become more easily recognizable. The easiest way to do this is to eat a meal or snack every 3–4 hours, while simultaneously checking in with the five areas where hunger can be detected – mood, energy, head, stomach, body. Go back to the hunger scan to help you.

If you experience chronic illness, or mental health issues, or require medication that alters how you experience physical sensations, I appreciate that it can be tricky to identify what is a real hunger signal. Repeating the hunger body scan practice above can help you get closer to deciphering what's what. You may also like to try following some gentle structure to recalibrate hunger and fullness signals. This might mean you aim to have 3 meals and 3 snacks at regular intervals, for example. I've worked with people who have more difficulty tuning into their bodies because of medical conditions, and although we can sometimes learn a lot from being curious about teasing apart hunger signals from the underlying condition, it's also not accessible to everyone all of the time. If this is you, remember you are not obligated to eat intuitively. Intuitive eating is a system of self-care: you can dip in and out of the elements that you find helpful, depending on your circumstances.

'Eat when hungry' isn't a rule!

Remember that getting familiar with your hunger signals isn't a mandate to 'only eat when you are hungry' – this is diet culture twisting things. Sometimes we need to eat when we're not hungry, for practical reasons. Like if you have three back-to-back meetings that go over lunch, you may want to have a snack beforehand so you don't perish in the middle of a presentation. Sometimes we might not be hungry in the moment but know if we wait until we can eat again we'll be overly hungry, and that will leave us feeling light-headed or nauseous, so it's better to plan ahead and have something to tide us over. Likewise, sometimes we end up going past the point of gentle hunger and into the overly hungry zone, not through choice, but because of our circumstances. This doesn't mean that you're 'failing' at intuitive eating (there is no failing, remember). But what can we learn from this experience for next time? Do we need to plan snacks better? Do we need to check in with our hunger cues more often? Be curious!

Keeping an intuitive eating journal

To help you notice patterns and get curious about your experiences with hunger signals (and later down the line, some of the other elements of intuitive eating), you can start keeping an intuitive eating journal. You can use the template in the appendix; remember, the intention is not to beat yourself up, but to gather data and information about your experiences. I usually recommend doing it for two or three days periodically throughout the process as a way of checking in with yourself. For some people this might feel a bit too much like tracking or food journaling – if that's you, don't worry about this activity. Otherwise, what information does journaling provide you with? Do you notice any patterns or trends? Are you routinely following hunger signals or do you get over-hungry regularly? Do your hunger signals change over the course of the day? Are they easier to tune into under different circumstances (for instance, at work vs at home or weekend vs weekday). Next, we will try and make sense of some of the information you've collected in your intuitive eating journal and help you interpret what it is telling us.

Interpreting your intuitive eating journal

To help you understand and connect with feelings of hunger, we can use the data you've collected in your intuitive eating journal and map it onto the hunger wheel. This can be particularly insightful if you're still struggling to connect with feelings of hunger, or if you find your critical voice judging you for how much/how often you're eating. I think it helps to visualize this, as just thinking about food can be a little nebulous.

So, in the appendix (page 313) there are some food icons for you to colour in and cut out. We will use these at different points in the book – so don't just skip over this part. It might seem like just a cutesy crafts project, but there is intention behind it.

Now we have our food icons ready to go, we can begin to map them across our day, comparing them with the hunger and satisfaction guide and our journal entries. So pick a day or two from your journal to focus on.

With your journal in front of you, use your food icons to visually represent each meal and snack you ate across the whole day.

* Arrange the food icons (by meal or snack), spreading them out to represent the time that has elapsed between each eating occasion. For example, if there was an hour between breakfast and morning snack, then it might be a smaller space. If there are 3 or 4 hours between eating, then the gap would be much bigger. This is to help you contextualize where food fits into your day, and identify any gaps where you may be going too long between eating, and therefore becoming over-hungry.

* Looking across the day, do you notice any large gaps between meals (how many hours?) where you may be more susceptible to becoming over-hungry? What impact did that have on your next meal or snack?

* Looking at the first thing you ate that day, what time did you go to bed the night before, and how long had it been since you last ate? How much sleep did you get, and did that impact your hunger? Did you eat close to waking up or was there a big gap, for example a commute to the office or a workout, before breakfast?

* How is your food spread across the day? Are your meals and snacks balanced over time or skewed towards the morning or evening?

* Reflecting on what you had at each eating occasion, was it a substantial meal or a smaller snack? Was it enough to keep you going to the next meal? I often ask clients, 'Was this enough food to feed a ten-year-old child?' If the answer is no, then it's definitely not enough for you!

* What were your hunger and fullness levels like around that meal? (Use the hunger wheel to help you determine this.)

* Had you done any exercise during that day or the day before? How might that have impacted your hunger?

Repeat this for all the meals and snacks you had throughout the day.

Reflecting back on your day, did you notice yourself judging your food choices? Weighing up how 'healthy' or 'unhealthy' they were? Are you berating yourself for not eating enough vegetables, or for having more than one serving of starchy food? Can you put all that to one side and just focus on whether or not you were eating enough throughout the day? Were you consistently honouring your hunger? Were you allowing yourself to fill up? Did you allow yourself regular snacks? Did the food icons and hunger scale corroborate one another?

In clinic I often notice that people have a tendency to 'backload' their eating. A helpful way to understand this is to imagine that first thing in the morning you totally drained your phone battery watching Instagram stories. You forget to take your charger with you and have to put your phone on low power mode. You steal little bits of juice from your friend's charger throughout the day, but never enough to fully power up, so you have to be super mindful of how you use your phone all day – no taking cute selfies, no FaceTiming your bestie, no firing off hilarious tweets, and worst of all, getting lost sans Google Maps. Your phone isn't firing on all cylinders. But then you get home at the end of the day and give it a full power-up. Right before bed. This is how we fuel our bodies. (Side note: full credit to Melanie on my team for this great analogy – thanks Mel!)

To help put this into perspective, a typical pattern I see is something a bit like this:

Exercising on an empty
stomach will cause the
tank to empty even further

Again I wonder if this
portion would be enough
to fill the tank all the
way to an 8!

Although this may have felt a bit chaotic and out
of control, this was probably a subjective binge
because 1) not enough food was eaten throughout
the day and 2) the foods that were eaten were all
relatively unexciting foods, meaning this person
probably felt a bit restricted and deprived and
craving something a bit more interesting to eat

Because of how long it had been between meals,
I wonder if this person was perhaps even lower on
the hunger scale than this! I expect they probably
weren't as full as this either, given that this
breakfast didn't have much substance to it.

	Time	What was eaten	Hunger	Fullness	Feeling	Time since last eaten
Dinner/snack (evening before)	8pm	Vegetable curry	2	8		3 hours
Sleep	11pm–6am		-	-		
Exercise (gym: treadmill and weights)	6:30am		5	5	Tired but need to go to gym	
Breakfast	9:30am (at desk)	Jam jar of overnight oats, tsp peanut butter, chia seeds, almond milk, blueberries	3	7		13 hours
Snack					Busy, stressed	
Lunch	1pm	Leftover vegetable curry	3	8		3.5 hours
Snack	5pm	Apple and peanut butter	2	6	Hassled at work	4 hours
Dinner	8pm	Smoked salmon, salad, baked sweet potato	1	5		3 hours
Snack	9pm	Cereal, peanut butter from jar, dark chocolate	7	10	Binge-y Feeling so guilty	

When we quantify it, 13 hours seems like a long time, but we don't often stop and notice how long it has been since we last ate – this can set us up to feel hungry and unsatisfied for the rest of the day

Based on your intuitive eating journal and the interpretation activity you have just completed, notice if your pattern of eating follows a similar trajectory. What would it be like to have a snack before the gym, or mid-morning? What would it be like to eat portions that are more closely aligned with our body's needs? Are the foods we select satisfying and interesting, or restrictive and likely to lead to intense cravings? If it's helpful, you could annotate your own intuitive eating journal using the prompts and questions above.

LEARNING TO TRUST OUR BODIES

There's a misconception that intuitive eating means simply 'listening to your body'. And while ultimately we do want to tune in more to what's going on below the neck, that doesn't mean we abandon our brain! We have been taught to *completely overthink* every decision around food, so that we end up getting stuck in our heads – just think back to the 'your brain on diets' activity in the last chapter. Intuitive eating invites us to find a semblance of balance between mind and body. The amount of headspace we dedicate to eating will fluctuate from person to person, and even for the same person from day to day. Sometimes we might need to give more thought and consideration to making sure we have stocked up on snacks and freezer meals. Other times we might have to make do with whatever we can get in the vending machine to fill a hole in our bellies, and pay little attention to our choices. None of this is right or wrong; this is flexible eating. But when we are completely disconnected from our bodies, we're more likely to be eating in a way that isn't satisfying and may even be disordered.

The difficulty is that many of us don't know *how* to trust our bodies to help guide our eating. I think this is one of the biggest things that people get stuck on when it comes to intuitive eating. We believe that intuitive eating means we have to trust our bodies, and we forget that *our bodies have to relearn how to trust us!* The relationship goes both ways. If we have been through prolonged periods of restriction and deprivation, short-changing our bodies, then why the hell would your body believe you when you say you're done with all that? It needs cold, hard evidence. In other words, in order for our bodies to believe us, we have to reliably and consistently (not just for a few days) give them regular, satisfying, enjoyable food. Only then will your body start to trust that you're not going to pull the rug out!

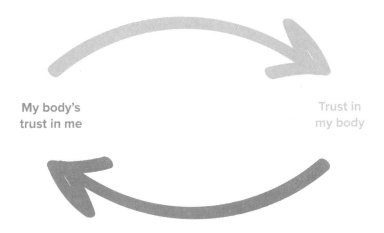

Learning to connect with and
understand my body's cues and signals

My body's
trust in me

Trust in
my body

Regular, adequate, sati,sfying, tasty meals and snacks

Rebuilding trust in our bodies can take time – remember back to how long you've been on a diet or restricting? (See your answer from page 79.) Now how long have you been learning about intuitive eating and how to honour your hunger? As well as eating regularly, we also have to be eating enjoyable and satisfying foods – we'll explore this more in Chapters 6 and 7.

In your journal, make a note of the answers to the following questions

+ What are your signals for hunger?

+ Have you been able to regularly check in with and act on your hunger signals?

+ What do you need to do to feel more confident leaning into these signals?

+ Have you noticed any fairy lights coming on?

+ Are there any tools from this section that you can add to your toolkit? Go back to Chapter 1 and write them in.

HOW TO JUST EAT IT

CHAPTER 4
BODY COMPASSION

Listen to the corresponding podcast episode Don't Salt My Game – How to Just Eat It: Chapter 4

I'm going to level with you. When it comes to cultivating better body image, I don't have any cute tricks. I don't know any magic formulas. There is no quick fix. What I do know is that the route of body shame lies in complicated cultural programming that needs to be brought to light, unpacked, and broken down. This is long, hard work – many entire books have been written on the topic – so consider this section a starting point to dig deeper. At the same time, there are practices we can cultivate to help us navigate body shame while we do all the unlearning. In this section we'll explore the cultural origins of body shame, and develop some practices to be kinder and gentler to your body and yourself as you dismantle what you have learned about your own and other people's bodies. To start with, it's helpful to examine the messages we've internalized about bodies: what constitutes a 'good' body and a 'bad' body, which bodies we find acceptable, and which we are repulsed by. All of this can give us clues about how to begin to unlearn our social conditioning about bodies.

> This section is safe for people with an eating disorder, although this can be very challenging if your eating disorder is very critical of your body. You may want to check in with your treatment team for support as you move through it.

'IDEAL' BODIES

Barbie dolls are some of the earliest role models that kids are exposed to and have been widely criticized for promoting highly unrealistic body ideals. For instance, in 1995 researchers found that in order for an average female body to meet the standards set out by Barbie dolls, they would need to grow 24 in. in height, increase their bust size by 5 in, increase neck length by 3.2 in., and lose 6 in. from the waist.[1] Now while Barbie isn't solely responsible for shaping body image in girls, her ubiquity makes her a meaningful contributor. So what happened when Mattel launched a new, curvier set of dolls? In 2019, body image researchers studied the impact that the new dolls had on young girls' body image.[2] Eighty-four girls aged between three and ten were given the classic doll (thin, white skin, blonde hair – you know what Barbie looks like!) or a new, curvier doll. The girls consistently attributed the original doll as being smart, happy, having friends, being pretty, and helping others. Whereas the curvy doll was considered to have no friends, not to be pretty, and to be mean; girls said they didn't want to play with this doll because she was 'big', 'fat', or 'chubby'. Now, my guess is that parents haven't been going around telling their kids that people in bigger bodies are mean and have no friends, but this is the subtext of a culture that values a particular body ideal over all else. We learn these messages by osmosis at a very, very young age, from the media, our parents, and even the toys we play with. Despite the fact that very few of us look like the cultural ideal (which would be biogenetically difficult, if not impossible for the vast majority of us!), we have internalized that as the gold standard with which we compare our bodies and other people's bodies too. It becomes the yardstick we use to measure our worth, and then beat ourselves up with when we fall short. Improving our body image has less to do with posting selfies in a bikini on Instagram and proclaiming our love for our bodies (that might be part of our process, and that's cool too); the real work is in uncovering our cultural programming and challenging our biases.

Radical self-love advocate and author of *The Body Is Not an Apology* (a must-read), Sonya Renee Taylor asks us to reflect on our cultural programming around bodies by inviting us to close our eyes and imagine a generic human to help us reveal the messages we have internalized about bodies. So, take a moment to close your eyes and let percolate for a second the thoughts, images, and ideas that come to mind when you imagine the quintessential human being. Notice their hair colour, eye colour, sound of their voice, height, size of their body, clothing, circumstances, and so on.

Use the following checklist to see how far your generic human strayed from the cultural size and beauty ideals we've inherited. How many of the following characteristics did your human have?

* White skin

* Young

* Blonde hair/blue eyes

* Able-bodied

* Thin (or Kardashian-esque 'curves-in-all-the-right-places')

* Muscular – '*Men's Health* cover star' type physique

* Cis-gendered

* Heterosexual

* Relatively affluent

* Native English speaker

* Did you imagine a Barbie doll???

For most of us, our minds will have gone to someone who looks a lot like the folks we see in the media: young, white, thin, attractive, rich, cis-gender, straight, and able-bodied. This becomes not only who we compare ourselves to, but also our standard of comparison for other people. If this is our default acceptable body, what does that mean for bodies that don't look like this ideal – the vast majority of people?

+ In what ways did your generic human match Eurocentric aesthetic ideals? In which way(s) did they deviate?

+ What can this activity tell you about how you've internalized cultural programming?

+ Which ways can you identify to begin to challenge this cultural programming?

+ When you are scrutinizing your body, can you gently remind yourself of your values?

WHAT'S THE STORY OF MY BODY?

In Chapter 2, we explored our relationship with food as we grew up and got more deeply entangled with diet culture. Now we're going to do something similar, except this time focusing on our bodies. The intention here is to explore how we have come to understand our bodies and the narrative we have created around them. This can be difficult and sometimes painful work, so if it feels too much, please do what you need to do to look after yourself. If you're really struggling, reach out for professional help if that's accessible to you.

In your journal, write or draw a timeline of your body, noticing salient events. You might like to zoom in on a specific period (pregnancy, puberty, getting married, divorced) or keep it looser and use major life milestones to jog your memory. The questions that follow will prompt you to reflect on these experiences.

* When did you first notice disliking your body or parts of your body?

* How were your parents'/caregivers' relationships with their bodies?

* What is your experience of being in your body?

* What makes you feel at home in your body?

* And what makes it feel uncomfortable or unsafe?

* What brings you joy and pleasure in your body?

* What messages did you receive about good and bad bodies?

* When have you felt gratitude and love towards your body?

* When have you felt discomfort or disdain for your body?

* What has your body allowed you to achieve or accomplish?

(Consider both the big things, like travel, education, having children, as well as little things like feeling the sun on our skin, holding loved ones, eating an incredible meal.)

* What has your body held you back from? How has it disappointed you?

* How has society informed you that you should view your body? Consider the following:

    - In what ways do you feel proud of your body?

    - What has diet culture and patriarchy taught you about your body?

    - How has fat phobia shaped how you see your body?

    - What has white supremacy and ableism taught you about your body?

    - How have heteronormative narratives influenced how you feel about your body?

    - How have your intersecting identities impacted on how you view your body?

By going through this activity, I hope you'll have a better awareness of how complex our relationships with our bodies are. It is rarely ever as simple as loving or hating your body; our bodies can be our homes and our sanctuaries, and at the same time they can feel like battlegrounds and carry enormous pain. Our bodies can do incredible things and are capable of surviving unthinkable trauma. By reflecting on our body stories, we can come to a new understanding and appreciation of them that has very little to do with our physical appearance. We can also begin to think of our bodies as companions that accompany us through life, carrying us, giving us a home, sharing our successes, and commiserating with us when things go wrong.

- Reflecting on your body story, has this changed the way you view your body?

- Have you been able to tap into gratitude, appreciation, or compassion for your body that you didn't have previously?

- If not, what steps could you take towards relating to your body differently?

- What scars or wounds do you think still need healing?

- How can you work towards this?

BODY NEUTRALITY

You've heard of body positivity, and I'm sure you're familiar with the idea of body hate (it's the air we breathe). Body neutrality is the idea that maybe we aren't totally comfortable with our bodies; we might be stuck in a place of cognitive dissonance, where we simultaneously understand that diets don't work, but are wrestling with wanting to change our bodies, and are still working towards unlearning our social programming and conditioning around bodies. This is totally understandable given how insidious diet culture is. But while you are working towards intuitive eating and ditching diet mentality, can you show your body some compassion and kindness? You may not love your body, and you may not even feel OK with your body, but can you show your body a level of care and decency that means it's getting its basic needs met?

This might look different for everyone, but here are some ideas for what body neutrality could look like:

* Regularly nourishing yourself with meals and snacks.

* Gentle movement that feels good in your body.

* Regular medical and dental check-ups.

* Taking care of your body (basic self-care, hygiene, taking medicines, sleep).

* Talking to your body with kindness.

* Practising self-compassion.

* Wearing clothes that are comfortable and don't rub, pinch, or dig.

* Seeking out pleasurable activities.

HOW TO JUST EAT IT

Here's what body neutrality is *not*:

* Restricting food, or dieting.

* Punishing yourself with exercise, or earning food through exercise.

* Pinching, poking, or otherwise being cruel to your body.

* Judging your own or other people's bodies.

* Body shaming (again, yourself or others).

* Taking things out on your body.

On our quest towards body neutrality, can we cultivate some compassion for our bodies? Before we go on to create our own body compassion practice, I want you to reflect on how you treat things you love versus things that you hate.

In your journal, write down what body compassion and body neutrality mean to you. How do they differ and how would you know if you were practising body compassion or body neutrality? What sort of things can you do to appreciate your body as it is now?

1. Think of an object, an item of clothing or furniture that you really dislike – how do you behave towards it? How do you touch it? How do you talk to/about it? What can this tell us about how we relate to our bodies? Can we notice when we're practising hatred towards them? And what would it feel like to be kinder?

2. How would you treat a person, pet, or a house plant that you really care about? How would you talk to them? How would you show love and kindness? How would you show compassion? How would they know they were valued and appreciated?

Sometimes it can be helpful to think of our bodies through a 'parenting' lens. There are times where we *just can't* with our kids, but would never dream of being cruel or unkind to them. We still provide them with all the ingredients they need to thrive and flourish.

Values and body compassion

How can you begin to see yourself as something worth caring for? Look back at your values list in Chapter 1 and think about how they can be used to guide you towards more body compassion. We tend to think of values as being directed outwards, but if they aren't directed back at ourselves, are we really tapping into their full potential? Granted they may not all apply to our bodies – but at least consider it! For instance, you may have creativity as one of your values. Can you channel that through experimenting with new clothes, nail art, or funky jewellery? Maybe one of your values is collaboration. How can you work with your body instead of against it? Or what if your value is fun? How can you have more fun in and with your body? That could be dancing or singing or having more sexy time.

Write out some ways you can experiment with channelling your values to show your body compassion

Value 1

How can I nurture this value in relation to my body?

Value 2

How can I nurture this value in relation to my body?

Value 3

How can I nurture this value in relation to my body?

Value 4

How can I nurture this value in relation to my body?

Value 5

How can I nurture this value in relation to my body?

Checking in with your values isn't something to be used for self-flagellation. It's an opportunity to check in with yourself, particularly when things feel difficult in and around your body.

Can you be curious about what might happen if you were to bring some of your values more into focus? What might be the result of embodying those values?

BUILD A BODY COMPASSION PRACTICE

Body compassion is a practice – that means setting aside deliberate, intentional time to commit to healing your relationship with your body. You might want to set aside some time each day, or a few days each week, whatever feels most supportive, to go through the steps you're going to set out for yourself – there will be times when you need it more than others, but it's helpful to practise when you're feeling OK, so that if things feel harder, these techniques feel safe and familiar. This practice might change over time, too, and you can update it as you find new tools, skills, and resources that feel supportive. Pick from the ideas listed here or come up with your own – many are from the toolkit, so head back to Chapter 1 to dust up on those skills.

Self-compassion practice (see Chapter 5, page 175)	Journaling (template in appendix, page 316)	Reading a chapter in a body liberation book
Anchoring	Listening to 30 minutes of a body liberation podcast	Meditation
Acceptance (listen to podcast from Chapter 1)	Checking in with body liberation activists on Instagram	Massaging a part of your body with kindness (and nice lotion)
Reading a poem about body compassion	Saying a mantra or affirmation	Looking at images of diverse bodies
Masturbation	Stretching or yoga	Checking in with my values

HOW TO JUST EAT IT

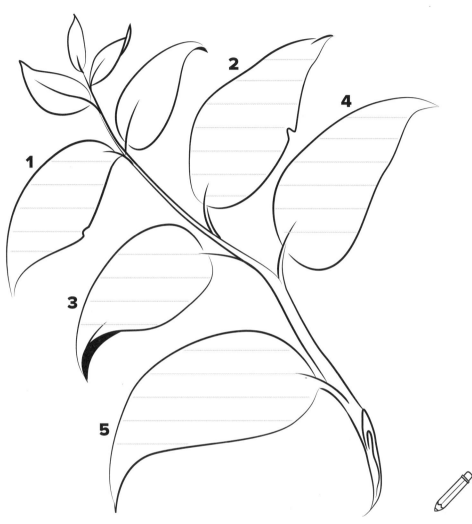

1

2

3

4

5

Write out your five-step body compassion practice in the spaces on this page, dedicating a new leaf to each step. Make this into a daily or weekly practice, to help foster body compassion

A LETTER TO MY BODY

Another way we can begin to develop body compassion is through writing a letter to our bodies. This can be a really cathartic, albeit challenging activity. The idea is to write either a letter of thanks and gratitude, a letter of apology for treating it badly, or perhaps one that encompasses both.

In your journal, try these written exercises.

1. Write an apology to your body for the years of abusive, punishing exercise, or the semi-starvation, for trying to squeeze it into clothes that don't fit, or for hating it for not fitting into society's narrow standards. This is obviously very difficult and potentially quite upsetting; if it feels too intense, then start with the second option.

2. Write a love letter to your body thanking it for all the incredible things it allows you to do, from moving through the world to allowing you to be intimate, to having children, swimming, dancing, reading, listening to music, hugging your dog, to just living and breathing.

> How did you find this activity? Was it challenging, cathartic, emotional? What did it bring up for you? What have you learned from it?

Exploring embodiment
(aka how to be more cat)

Nicola Haggett
Certified body trust
provider & intuitive
eating coach
@nicolahaggett

Embodiment is one of those concepts that sounds cool but is a bit hard to get your head around. There are lots of definitions out there, but for me, the one that resonates most is the experience of feeling 'at one' or 'at home' in your body (rather than living 'from the head up').

Easier said than done, you might say.

As a fat person, I've spent most of my adult life trying to shrink my body in order to fit in. So the idea of feeling 'at home' in my body (without trying to change it first) used to sound like a tall order; that kind of thing was reserved for 'after'. After I lost weight, after I fixed my body image, after I'd tried harder.

But it hasn't always been that way. We are born into this world feeling 'at home' in our bodies. It's our birthright. I remember gleefully powering around on my roller-skates as a kid, marvelling at the power in my legs. Free from judgement or shame about my body.

But then, somewhere along the way, that sense of positive embodiment got hijacked by the messages I absorbed as I grew up. Messages about what it meant to be a 'good' girl, and the ideals I internalized about the kinds of bodies that were 'good', 'healthy', 'worthy'. And how my body did, or didn't, measure up to that.

We live in a culture that conditions us to leave our body. It tells us we constantly need to be working on our bodies, fixing them, in an endless self-improvement project. Disconnection through dieting, numbing, overworking becomes our way to find relief from never feeling quite good enough.

So how do we start to reclaim a sense of feeling more at home in our bodies? This question's even trickier to answer because we live in a culture that makes it harder for some bodies (such as fat, queer, BAME, disabled, or older bodies) to move through the world than others.

Dr Niva Piran (a super cool feminist psychologist, researcher, and activist) did some interesting research into the quality of girls' and women's experiences of being in their bodies, across different stages in their lives (their 'body journeys'). From this research, she derived the Developmental Theory of Embodiment (DTE), which explores the ways in which social powers and privilege impact our experiences of embodiment.[3]

One entry point into reclaiming your body as your home might be to explore your own 'body journey'. Think back to how you used to feel in your body, and consider how you feel in your body today. What journey has your body been on? To find out, make a timeline, grab a journal, or bust out your art supplies. Consider the following:

✖ What's come between you and being in your body?
✖ What social and cultural conditions have enhanced or disrupted your ability to trust your body?
✖ When did you first learn that your body was a problem?

Through this process, you might find that you can start to shift some of the anger and shame you have internalized towards your body, and start to direct it, more appropriately, at the external sources of that pain.

It was never your fault. Your body was never the problem.

Next, look for ways to enhance your experiences of embodiment intentionally, to connect to and listen to your body – despite living in a society that doesn't always make this easy.

But where to start?

In her research, Dr Piran proposes that we experience embodiment across five different dimensions:

* Body connection and comfort
* Agency and functionality
* Experience and expression of desires
* Attuned self-care
* Inhabiting the body as a subjective site (resisting objectification)

Academic research can sometimes feel a bit 'heady' and hard to put into practice (no offence to any academics out there!). So when I was trying to find ways to explore the Developmental Theory of Embodiment in my own life, I looked around for positive role models of embodiment across all five dimensions . . . and I drew a bit of a blank.

That's where my neighbour's cat comes in — casually stretched across the lawn, basking in the sunlight, taking up space, and giving no f**ks about the fact that this is my garden, not his. I wished I could be more like him.

I looked at Dr Piran's framework from the perspective of a cat, and it turns out they are actually pretty cool representations of embodiment!

Body connection and comfort: Cats have a natural sense of pride, of knowing that their body is 'good'. They seek out places and people that make them feel safe and comfortable. They know that they deserve to be treated with respect and care at all times.

Agency and functionality: Cats like their freedom. They like to come and go as they please, and aren't afraid to take up space (even if they aren't in their own garden).

Experience and expression of desires: Cats are very clear about who has consent to stroke them, pet them, and pick them up. They offer up affection (purrrrrr) and engage in playtime on their terms, not anyone else's.

Attuned self-care: Cats are good at listening to their bodies. They nap when they need to, communicate their feelings, seek out food when they're hungry, and have clear boundaries (hisssss!).

Inhabiting the body as a subjective site (resisting object-ification): Cats don't need to worry about what others are thinking about their body. They move to serve a purpose, or in a way that feels good. They seek out places where they can move out of a sense of empowerment: to pounce, play, hide, or nap.

So, when I want to practise embodiment, I find somewhere quiet, check in with my body, and channel my Inner Cat. What's here? What sounds good? What do I need more of, less of, right now?

Maybe I want to put on something soft and cosy. Maybe I need to stretch. Maybe I want to seek out my partner's touch, or a friend's company. Maybe I want to engage in some positive self-talk. Maybe I want to be on my own. Maybe I want some yummy food. Maybe I am feeling playful and 'pouncy', and I want to go for a walk. Maybe I need to have a word with someone who's crossed my boundaries.

The more you practise being 'Cat', the easier it becomes. Give it a go! It's a fun and gentle way to start exploring embodiment, showing your body that it's worthy of care, worthy of paying attention to, and that you can trust it (and yourself). It's a way to come 'home'.

✚ What does the term embodiment mean to you?

✚ Do you tend to spend more time with your thoughts and feelings ('in your head'), or do you have a practice of checking in with your body regularly? If not, what gets in the way?

✚ Diet culture, fat phobia, and other systems of suppression teach us to override signals and messages from our bodies. What are some ways you have been taught to ignore your body?

✚ What do you notice about the quality of your experiences of embodiment across the five dimensions from Dr Piran's research? Which area do you feel strongest in? Which area would benefit from some attention and practice?

✚ Can you think of a role model that comes to mind when you think of positive embodiment? If the example of a cat doesn't resonate with you, what might? When it comes to giving some attention and practice to one of the five dimensions of embodiment, practise checking in with that role model – what are they inviting you to experiment with?

✚ Many (but not all) of us had more positive experiences of embodiment as children. When you think back, can you remember an example of feeling 'at home' in your body, perhaps during a carefree moment or when playing? How does that differ from your experience of your body now?

✚ Dr Piran's research talks about how social and cultural conditions, as well as our identities, impact our experiences of embodiment. Can you think of any ways they have enhanced your experiences of embodiment? Can you think of any ways they have made it harder for you to feel 'at home' in your body?

+ Thinking about your own body journey, what stories about your body have you been carrying that don't belong to you? Can you acknowledge that they were never yours in the first place? What does it open up for you to do so?

+ What kind of relationship with your body would you love to live your way into?

THINKING BEYOND OUR
OWN EXPERIENCES

The following guest essay from comedian Sofie Hagen speaks to the fact that cultivating a personal body compassion practice doesn't reduce the harm that is inflicted on bodies at a broader societal level. Almost all bodies experience oppression as a result of the cultural beauty standard. Even if you fit these ideals, what is the cost of maintaining them? And what is the cost if you don't? But the more you 'deviate' from these ideals – the bigger, the fatter your body – the more privilege you lose. You are pushed farther towards the margins. You experience more bigotry, discrimination, hatred, injustice, and prejudice. This is why the fat activism movement pushes for equality and justice for all bodies, including those that society as a whole deems 'unworthy'. Many of us don't stop to consider what it might feel like to be told our body is an 'epidemic', a drain on public health resources, or to be verbally and physically abused because of our body size, because many of us never have to experience it. Although the majority of us have experienced the oppression of the patriarchy and diet culture, it is a minority of us who have had to live in a world that hates us and reminds us daily that it does not want us in it. I hope Sofie's essay gives some insight into the experience of fatness – and makes clear that no amount of self-love can undo systemic fat phobia. I also hope that it acts as a reminder for those of us with thin privilege to speak up when we see and hear fat phobia in action – this does not mean speaking over or for fat people, but disrupting the dominant narrative that fat is bad, ugly or unhealthy. Call out your friends and family when they make a fat joke. Challenge brands that have a size limit on clothes or products. Demand media outlets don't use offensive language (like ob*se) or imagery (like headless fat bodies) to describe fat bodies. Most importantly, listen to fat people, follow them on social media, and support their work.

Sofie Hagen
Comedian, author of
Happy Fat and host of the
Made of Human podcast
@sofiehagendk

Fat accessibility

I am a nervous flyer. This has nothing to do with fearing a plane crash. More often than not, I am in so much physical and emotional pain on planes that I would welcome some turbulence, just for the distraction. At the time of writing this, I am six months away from my next flight – and I think about it once a week. My heart starts pounding, my palms are sweaty. What if the price goes up so much that I won't be able to afford two seats? What if, when I call them, they won't allow me to buy two seats? What if someone takes my photo and posts it on their Instagram with the caption 'when you're sitting next to an actual whale on your flight'? What if I have to sit in tremendous pain for hours and hours, again?

On a flight from England to Australia a couple of years ago, right before they closed the doors, two teenage boys got on and took the two seats next to me, their entire demeanour very obviously noticing my size. They spoke in a language I didn't understand – and while I didn't know any of the words, I have had my fatness mocked my entire life, and I know how it sounds. The tone, the disgust, the hand gestures, the glances. I pressed my thighs together, hard; twisted my upper body sideways, so my shoulder was pressed against the window and my knees against the wall. Every time a piece of my flesh touched the boy next to me, he recoiled and said something to his friend, who then looked at me. When the food came, a few hours into the fourteen-hour flight from Dubai to Melbourne, I said 'no thanks'. There was not enough room for the tray table because of my stomach. And even if I wanted to eat, I would have to use both hands, meaning I'd have to sit up straight, not crouched with my shoulders pushed together, and then I would be in the way for the boy sitting next to me. The armrest was already pressing into my flesh. Twelve hours to go.

HOW TO JUST EAT IT

There are bars I have had to leave because I couldn't physically fit into the bathroom stall and onto the toilet. Usually I just have half a butt resting on a sanitary bin, and I need to do advanced acrobatics to find a way to wipe myself. If you invite me out for dinner, I will spend hours finding a place that has a big enough gap between the tables, so that my stomach won't fling someone's chicken off their plate as I try to get by. Any chair with armrests is a no-go, and I will have to ask a waiter if they have a different one, and they will look me up and down and sigh – or even worse, they will tear up and feel pity for me. Seats in general, of course, are the enemy of the fat. Planes, trains, buses, cinemas, cafés, hairdressers, and so on. On average, there are four seats in a standard theatre that I can fit into – and they are hundreds of pounds more expensive than the rest, and I need to book them months in advance. I cried through *Hamilton*, like everyone else, but for a different reason: the seats had cut off blood to my legs and it hurt.

And those are just the physical limits.

When I need to see a medical professional, I get immediate anxiety. I know they will want to weigh me. I know they won't take me seriously. I know they will suggest that I lose weight or even offer me weight-loss surgery. I know that I will not receive the same care that a smaller person would. I know all of the stories and statistics. The GP is always shocked when my blood pressure is fine and I don't present with diabetes. They always suggest that I go for a walk every morning and that I eat less pasta. As if I have never heard of the idea of carbs and exercise. Like that's the reason I'm fat: that I just didn't know that choc-olate wasn't slimming.

I don't go to nightclubs or bars on the weekends because 'fuck a pig' is a popular game among certain groups of men; they compete to see who can get the fat girl's attention, and then mock her for falling for it. Sometimes you're just invisible for the night. You're not a romantic or sexual option. You're just in the way. Dating sites and apps are off the table. Men will purposely swipe right just to let you know you are too fat.

Say I want to start working out. The gym is inherently unsafe: I have seen hundreds of candid photos of fat people on treadmills with some hilarious caption underneath, mocking them. Besides, there are fat-phobic messages everywhere. I could, of course, just exercise at home – if it wasn't for the fact that most exercise equipment has a weight limit way below what I weigh.

And say I needed to buy gym clothes first – or just clothes in general. Show me a physical store where I can buy clothes that fit me. I have not bought clothes in a physical shop since 2001. Even clothing brands that pride themselves on having plus-size collections don't stock it in the actual physical stores, unless it's in a pile in the corner. 'ONE SIZE FITS ALL' means 'unless you're fat'. 'ALL SIZES' means 'up to a size 22, at best'.

For me, being fat means a whole lot of anxiety, stress, and having to spend a lot of money just to avoid physical pain from various seats. Despite all of this, I consider myself lucky. I'm lucky because I sometimes have the money. I'm lucky because I am the one whose words you're reading. But for people who do not have the luxury of disposable income – or the people who are fatter than me, for whom the world is even less accessible – this brief essay would sound very different. It would mean never eating out, never travelling, never getting to exercise, never going to the theatre or the cinema, never going to bars or night-clubs, never having a way to try and find love or sex, and never going to the doctor's, even if they are sick. Many fat people don't even have the privilege of being in intense pain, just so they can see Australia or *Hamilton*.

In your journal, answer the following questions.

1. How has your body size made it easier or less easy to move through the world?

2. How has your size impacted how people treat you?

3. Do you feel that everyone should have the same access to theatre, travelling, and restaurants?

**Jess Campbell BSc,
PgDip, Current
Candidate MBChB**
Non-diet nutritionist
and medical student,
and campaigner
for weight-inclusive
healthcare practices
@haes_studentdoctor

Health At Every Size®

You might have picked this book up because you're questioning the way we talk about weight and health. A personal experience with chronic dieting may have you wondering if the problem with diets is really your fault or if it was the dieting all along! Or perhaps you are a health professional and recognize that despite best efforts to be helpful, weight management conversations undermine the therapeutic relationship. You may be noticing that weight loss attempts, followed by weight cycling and the impact of weight stigma are indeed more harmful than helpful in the long term.

Weight has long been used as a proxy for a person's health status and has become a measure of apparent engagement in health or so-called lifestyle behaviours – such as the frequency of exercise and the amount or quality of food consumed. A person's weight is frequently used as a 'clue' for a range of other physical, psychological, social, and character assumptions we make about one another – whether it be a tendency toward mental health concerns such as depression and anxiety, perhaps a history of trauma, or that a fat body equates to a gluttonous or lazy personality.

As a health professional I'm educated to use a person's weight in determining a risk profile for developing disease and to seek weight reducing measures to attend to these risks. Despite this being the conventional approach in health and medical practice, it's become increasingly evident that body weight as an indicator of health is not particularly helpful; nor is it supported by robust evidence and certainly not by the experiences of patients.

The association of body weight with health outcomes is complex, and there are very few conditions where a causal relationship has been established, despite what explosive media headlines report. The premise of weight reduction as an appropriate intervention for any risk associated with high body mass index (BMI) is flawed, for two main reasons. Firstly, we remain unable to produce evidence that we can consistently, effectively and safely affect body size and maintain weight losses over the long term; however, evidence to the contrary continues to grow. Secondly, we simply do not know if reducing a person's body weight confers a risk reduction compared to having never been at a higher weight to begin with. Prescribing weight loss to reduce risk is not data driven: the evidence doesn't exist, because there aren't enough folks who have sustained meaningful weight loss to study in order to adequately answer that question. Weight loss recommendations are often based on 'clinical experience' and 'expert consensus' – and what this really means is 'assumption'.

Over half a century ago, fat activists and scholars presented critical analysis of the research connecting higher weight with poor health. Today, this body of work and information remains just as relevant, and apparently difficult to move into mainstream medicine and health care provision. The global 'obesity epidemic' messaging strengthens and we continue to work with a predominantly weight normative model of care.

Weight normative care centres body weight and weight management as a core determinant of health and wellbeing, with an emphasis on engaging in weight reducing methods to achieve a 'healthy' weight – typically determined by the 'normal' range of BMI.

The missed opportunity in this conventional approach is in understanding and addressing the impact of the social determinants of health – these are the big picture influences: access to appropriate and timely health care, employment, education and economic opportunities, the environment in which we live, access to natural resources, our social connections, and safety for ourselves and the communities with which we identify. It's a lot to sideline when caring for humans – the concept of health and health care of the physical body alone is very limited, our wellbeing is influenced by our experiences and interactions with socio-political systems as we move about the world.

In Australia there have been encouraging developments, with both the Royal Australasian Colleges for Physicians (RACP) and General Practitioners (RACGP) have made recommendations that health professionals reorient practice from weight loss towards health gain. These organizations recognize that lifestyle and behaviour interventions for weight loss are ineffective, and not without risk of psychological and physical harm for some patients. This shift in focus from weight loss to health gain also recognizes that the prescription of weight management advice has continued to perpetuate weight stigma, shame and avoidance of health care.

Health at Every Size® (HAES) is an international movement with philosophical principles that offer a framework and structure for health care practitioners to deliver and patients to access affirming, informed care that seeks health gain without the pursuit of weight loss. The HAES philosophy affirms a broad, holistic definition of health – not restricted to the absence of disease – and that the concept of 'health' be a self-defined capacity or resource available to all irrespective of one's health status and ability. Its set of principles developed by health care practitioners, consumers and activists who reject the use of BMI and weight as proxies for health, that weight status is indicative of intention or engagement in health behaviours, and that there is significant 'controllability' of body weight, offers an approach to individual and community health via policy and individual decision-making processes.

These are the principles as outlined by the The Association for

Size Diversity and Health (ASDAH) who are committed to HAES principles:

* **Weight inclusivity** Accept and respect the inherent diversity of body shapes and sizes and reject the idealizing or pathologizing of specific weights.

* **Health enhancement** Support health policies that improve and equalize access to information and services, and personal practices that improve human wellbeing, including attention to individual physical, economic, social, spiritual, emotional, and other needs.

* **Respectful care** Acknowledge our biases, and work to end weight discrimination, weight stigma, and weight bias. Provide information and services from an understanding that socio-economic status, race, gender, sexual orientation, age, and other identities impact weight stigma, and support environments that address these inequities.

* **Eating for wellbeing** Promote flexible, individualized eating based on hunger, satiety, nutritional needs, and pleasure, rather than any externally regulated eating plan focused on weight control.

* **Life-enhancing movement** Support physical activities that allow people of all sizes, abilities, and interests to engage in enjoyable movement, to the degree that they choose.

There is a growing scientific evidence base examining the psychological and biomedical efficacy of HAES care. To summarize, HAES interventions have been found to sustain health-supporting eating habits and improve a range of psychological outcomes, including improved body image and self-esteem, and reductions in internalized weight stigma. Biomedical outcomes associated with HAES care when compared to conventional weight loss trials include similar reductions in cardiovascular health indices such as blood pressure and cholesterol – importantly, this finding demonstrates that health gains can be achieved independent of weight loss.

Progress is slow, but we are beginning to see a mainstream interest in weight inclusive care across a range of health practitioner codes. Psychotherapy and dietetics have made significant inroads in both professional practice and teaching programmes across the USA, Australia and New Zealand. Medicine, nursing and allied health practitioners are beginning to assimilate HAES practices as demand increases and the benefits become increasingly evident. I am hopeful that we are riding a groundswell of change that would lead to these practices becoming integral in health care provision. From this vantage point we can look back at the ripples that created this movement, the decades of labour by fat activists and clinicians, and look forward to changing the conversations we are having about health, weight, and bodies.

If you were to zoom the lens out on the concept of health, how would you define it...

+ for yourself?

+ for your family?

+ for your community or a community you identify with?

Note down a few things you can do today to move towards self-defined health or health values.

Are there any health practices that are no longer serving you?

Create an elevator pitch for how you would explain a weight inclusive approach to health to someone who has never heard of the concept before.

What are three things you'd like your doctor to know when caring for you?

+ Have any fairy lights turned on for you in this section?

+ What have I learned about how I treat my body? How has this been influenced by diet culture and fat phobia?

+ What messages have I internalized about 'good' and 'bad' bodies?

+ Which of these pieces resonate for you? What have you learned about other people's experiences with body compassion and the challenges in accessing it?

+ Are there any tools from this section that you can add to your toolkit? Go back to Chapter 1 and write them in.

Listen to the corresponding podcast episode Don't Salt My Game – How to Just Eat It: Chapter 5

CHAPTER 5

UNDERSTANDING EMOTIONAL EATING

Depending on the eating disorder, you may turn more to restriction when you're dealing with uncomfortable feelings. These activities can help you learn new or different ways of coping that don't rely on eating disorder behaviours, but if in doubt, talk to your treatment team.

In the context of diet culture, eating to soothe emotions is a big NO-NO. It's become vilified, and if you google 'emotional eating' you'll get sent to all kinds of weight-loss apps and 'how-to-stop' guides. It becomes another aspect of eating that we need to have control and dominance over, instead of responding with curiosity and non-judgement. What if we reframed it? Let's consider what emotional eating has done to help you. I know that might sound weird at first. But here's the thing. If emotional eating wasn't serving an important purpose, you'd have ditched it by now, right? Emotional eating isn't inherently bad. It might have been the best we could do at the time to deal with whatever difficult or challenging things were going on in our lives: a coping mechanism which might actually give us some clues and insight into unmet needs.

In your journal, write out all the functions that food has served over the years that you have labelled as 'emotional', 'stress', or 'comfort' eating.

Use the following for inspiration:

numbing out	pacifying feelings of shame
distraction	ignoring feelings of agitation
comfort	squashing embarrassment
contentment	dealing with loneliness
self-soothing	celebration
neutralizing overwhelm	joy
calming restlessness	excitement

Next to each one, write down any associations or memories you have with food. Did this give you any clues as to your own unmet needs?

Could it be you're simply hungry?

You might want to take a seat, because what I'm about to say might just blow your mind. Sometimes what we label 'emotional eating' is actually just hunger! We talked about the idea of backloading meals and the potential problems that can cause in Chapter 3; I'm reiterating it here because I see it happen time after time in clinic. Clients don't offer themselves enough nourishment to get through the day, so by the time they get home in the evenings they feel compelled to eat whatever they can get their paws on. Then that judgey voice in our heads labels it 'emotional' or 'comfort' eating, which it also judges as 'bad'. This can so easily trigger a compensatory behaviour, such as restriction or over-exercising, which will only exacerbate the cycle of binge/restrict and strengthen that critical voice. If you're not sure if you're eating enough throughout the day, it can sometimes be worth adding a morning or afternoon snack to see if this helps abate some of the evening fridge raids. If it doesn't, then that gives you a clue that there's something else going on.

OK, so you're eating enough – now check in with your self-care

When our self-care is 'off' it can lead to disruptions in our ability to respond to our internal cues, our *interoceptive awareness*. Things that throw off our interoceptive awareness are called 'attunement disruptors'. Basically, they make it hard to perceive the other sensations in our body.

You'll know this yourself: when you haven't had enough sleep, the next day you might feel extra hungry, or make food choices that don't help you feel your best. Likewise, some people don't feel hunger when they're stressed out and might end up under-eating in response. Listen, I get it: 'self-care' has become this super annoying, Instagram aspirational, bubble baths and pedicures bullshit. And while those things are great, what I'm talking about here is basic. It's ensuring that we're looking out for our physical and emotional well-being, and our mental health.

SELF-CARE ASSESSMENT

The following chart is a self-care assessment adapted from one developed by researcher Catherine Cook-Cottone.[1] It divides self-care up into six domains: supportive structure, mindful relaxation, self-compassion and purpose, mindful and non-judgemental awareness, supportive relationships, and physical care. These are the areas that Catherine's research has identified as being important to holistic self-care; notice how different that is from diet culture's idea of self-care, which is essentially: 'eat green things, do loads of workouts, maybe meditate'.

Take some time to go through the self-care assessment, checking the statements you agree with. Note that the operative word here is assessment, not checklist or to-do list. It's an opportunity to check in with yourself and notice the areas you might not be getting enough self-care in. It's not an invitation to berate yourself for 'failing', but a chance to bring awareness to things you might not have otherwise considered or perhaps pushed down because they felt too tough to deal with.

Supportive practices

Supportive structure	Mindful relaxation	Self-compassion and purpose	Mindful and non-judgey awareness	Supportive relationships	Physical care
☐ I keep my work/ study areas organized to support me	☐ I do something intellectual to help me relax (read a book, write a journal, do puzzles)	☐ I'm OK with my own challenges and difficulties	☐ I have mindful, non-judge-mental awareness of my thoughts	☐ I spend time with people who are good to me (support, encourage, believe in me)	☐ I drink enough water
☐ I maintain a manageable schedule	☐ I do something interpersonal to relax (chill with friends or family – IRL or virtually)	☐ I don't trash-talk myself ('I'm doing the best I can')	☐ I have mindful, non-judge-mental awareness of my feelings	☐ I feel supported by people in my life	☐ I eat regular meals and snacks
☐ I maintain a balance between the demands of others and what is important to me	☐ I do something creative to relax (draw, play music, write creatively)	☐ I remind myself that shit hitting the fan is a normal part of being a human	☐ I have mindful, non-judge-mental awareness of my body	☐ I have someone I can call when I'm upset	☐ I move my body in a way that feels joyful
☐ My home environment is comfortable and welcoming	☐ I listen to relax (to music, a podcast, radio show, audiobook)	☐ I allow myself to feel my feelings (e.g. I allow myself to cry)	☐ I carefully select which of my thoughts and feelings I use to guide my actions	☐ I feel confident that people in my life would respect my choice to say 'no'	☐ I make time for rest
	☐ I seek out images to relax (art, film, nature, Netflix)	☐ I experience meaning and/or purpose in my work/student life (e.g. it's for a cause or the greater good)		☐ I schedule time to be with people who are special to me	☐ I get adequate sleep to feel rested and restored
	☐ I seek out smells to relax (nature, candles, aromatherapy, cooking/ baking)	☐ I experience meaning and/or purpose in my private/personal life (e.g. for a cause)			☐ If I am unwell, I visit my doctor or take time off work

Self-care disruptors

Supportive structure	Mindful relaxation	Self-compassion and purpose	Mindful and non-judgey awareness	Supportive relationships	Physical care
☐ My living space is disorganized and chaotic	☐ I don't allow myself any downtime	☐ I'm very hard on myself and rarely give myself a break	☐ I am judgemental of my thoughts	☐ My friends are emotional vampires (they suck my energy and leave me drained)	☐ I don't drink enough water
☐ I overschedule and overcommit myself	☐ I don't know how to relax	☐ I have negative self-talk	☐ I am judgemental of my feelings		☐ I regularly skip meals and snacks
☐ I let other people dictate my schedule	☐ I feel as though I always have to be productive	☐ I have to do everything perfectly and if something goes wrong it means I've failed	☐ I am judgemental of my body	☐ I don't feel supported by the people in my life	☐ I use exercise as a form of punishment/ compensation or avoid it altogether
☐ I am a people pleaser and too often put my needs second	☐ I have a tough time managing stress		☐ I make decisions without checking in with my thoughts and feelings	☐ I don't have anyone to call when I'm upset	☐ I feel guilty for resting
	☐ I regularly want to zone out and avoid real life*	☐ I push my feelings down and try to ignore them		☐ People in my life don't respect my boundaries	☐ I don't get enough sleep to feel rested and restored
		☐ My work/ student life doesn't fulfil me		☐ I don't prioritize spending time with people who are special to me	☐ If I am unwell, I keep pushing through instead of taking time off
		☐ My personal life doesn't fulfil me		☐ I withdraw from people when I'm stressed out	

*Sometimes you need to check out after a stressful day and that's totally normal and can be part of self-care. What we mean here is more a habitual zoning out so you don't have to deal with real life

UNDERSTANDING EMOTIONAL EATING

Increasing self-care practices

 Using the self-care assessment tool, review the different categories of self-care in your journal and think about which ones you might like to focus on increasing.

Describe one or two strategies for each category that you would like to consistently practise to support your self-care. Make sure these are realistic – don't go from 0 to 100 if that is actually going to cause more stress!

Supportive structures: I'll turn down any new volunteer commitments until my current ones have ended

Mindful relaxation: I'll spend twenty minutes reading my book when I get home from work on two days this week

Self-compassion and urpose: I'll listen to a 5-minute self-compassion meditation in the morning

Mindful, non-judgey awareness: I'll practise putting negative thoughts about my body back on the sushi train

Supportive relationships: I'll spend time with a friend this weekend by planning a coffee date

Physical care: I'm going to make a bedtime routine and try to get to sleep by 10:30pm

> + What challenges or obstacles are in the way of tending more to my self-care needs?
>
> + Is it possible for me to reduce or remove these obstacles?
>
> + Have I noticed a correlation between not meeting my self-care needs and using food to soothe difficult feelings?

IDENTIFYING PHYSICAL VS EMOTIONAL HUNGER

By now you probably understand the signs and symptoms of physical hunger, but just in case, here's a recap.

Physical hunger symptoms

* builds gradually

* accompanied by low energy, low mood, lack of concentration or dull headache, rumbling sensations in your belly, and/or a weak feeling in your body

* satisfied by eating something

* you may be irritable (again relieved by eating)

* time has passed since your last meal or snack

We also experience something called 'taste hunger', which is the sensation that you want to eat something just because you like the taste of it. This is usually satisfied by having a couple of spoonfuls of Nutella or peanut butter, a few handfuls of crisps, or a bowl of ice cream, a few slices of cheese, that sort of thing. If you feel as though you need a much larger amount of food to satisfy that craving, then you might be looking at emotional hunger. Just a small caveat here – even if we are eating *regularly* and eating *enough*, if you're not eating satisfying foods and are still restricting, this could be contributing to a sense of emotional eating – we'll unpack this more in Chapter 8: Mindful Eating and Finding Pleasure in Food.

Emotional hunger symptoms

* no physical hunger cues – but other bodily sensations might provide clues as to your feelings or needs

* very specific cravings that aren't satisfied when you eat what you're craving (side note: cravings on their own are common and not necessarily connected to emotional eating)

* food doesn't completely satisfy, no matter how much you eat

* occurs shortly after your last meal or snack

* looking aimlessly in fridge/kitchen

So, if you've identified that you're 100 per cent *not* physically hungry, it's not taste hunger, and that no amount of food will fill you up, then it's likely that you're experiencing emotional hunger. The tricky part now is identifying what you're feeling. This can be tough if we're used to eating our emotions and trying to stuff them down instead of feeling them.

EMOTIONS WORD WHEEL

One way to try and connect with how we're feeling is to identify and name those emotions, using the Emotions Word Wheel tool. It's often easier to identify one of the six emotions in the middle of the wheel and then work outwards to narrow it down into more nuanced descriptions.

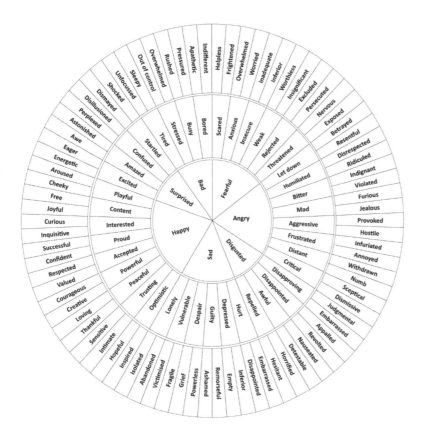

Using colouring pens or pencils, shade in the colours you associate with each feeling; the intensity of the shading can represent how strongly you feel that emotion

Which feelings tend to come up for you in relation to food (by which I mean which feelings tend to come up for you *before* you eat for emotional relief, as opposed to how you feel about eating, i.e. guilty)?

UNDERSTANDING EMOTIONAL EATING   **161**

* In the outer wheel, can you notice which foods you eat in relation to that emotion?

* Is there any relationship between the foods you eat around difficult or upsetting emotions, versus those that are perhaps considered more positive or happy emotions?

* Can you also begin to identify what else can meet that need? What self-care practices might you find helpful and soothing? (You can annotate this on the wheel to help you identify it at times where you might be struggling!)

Often there's an overlap with the types of foods we eat for celebration, fun, pleasure, joy and play, and those we eat for comfort, reassurance, and soothing. What does this tell us about what might be going on for us? Are we trying to elicit the same feelings we associate with happiness when we turn to celebration or comforting foods during times of stress? I don't know that there's any hard data on this, but my sense is that we gravitate towards pleasurable foods to conjure up those feelings of warmth and comfort. Sometimes the food might be just what we need, other times it might be something else. A lot of the time it's both!

UNDERSTANDING FEELINGS IN THE BODY

Back in Chapter 3 when we talked about interoceptive awareness, we saw how feelings and emotions originate in the body, and then get interpreted by the brain (granted that sometimes our brain has no idea how to make sense of them!).

Researchers have tried to capture this phenomenon using a bodily sensations map.[2] These are subjective depictions of where different emotions and physical states occur in the body, and can be helpful if you're out of touch with how emotions manifest themselves physically. But of course, it's limited. For example, as we've already discussed, hunger can show up in lots of places in the body besides the stomach, but the depiction here is mainly in the belly and a little in the head. So while I think it's pretty cool to look at (and might give us some insight into our own experiences), it can be a good idea to create our own subjective bodily sensations map or maps. Doing it yourself means you can also add more detail to help reflect how exactly it shows up for you! Here are a few examples of feelings and sensations, you can access the full map by searching online for 'bodily sensations map' and clicking on images.

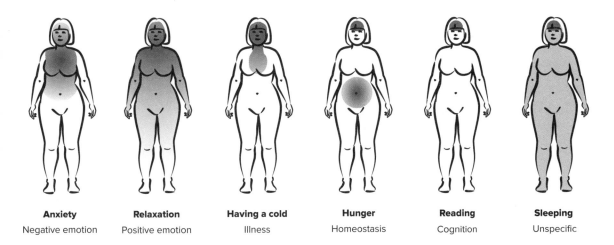

| **Anxiety** | **Relaxation** | **Having a cold** | **Hunger** | **Reading** | **Sleeping** |
| Negative emotion | Positive emotion | Illness | Homeostasis | Cognition | Unspecific |

Think about whereein your body you're experiencing an emotion. There's no need to name it yet, just think about how it feels in the body. There may be multiple emotions present at the same time, so you can either map them on the same figure or make copies for each emotion.

For each sensation, think about the following characteristics:

Physical location: head, heart, chest, stomach, shoulders, neck, jaw, lungs, etc

Shape: circle, triangle, amorphous blob, squiggle, spiral, zigzag, octagon, etc

Colour: choose a colour that best reflects the emotion

Size: how intensely you're feeling the emotion might be reflected in its size

Patterns or textures: ridges, bumps, smoothness, checks, swirls, spikes, etc

Once you've determined the form the emotion has taken, draw it on the figure opposite. Now you can see a visual representation of your emotion, can you give it a name using the emotion wheel? Are you able to identify the trigger for the emotion? Can you identify what purpose food might be serving to soothe that emotion? Does this give you any clues as to what you need, and how to meet that need?

Next time you're experiencing an uncomfortable emotion and find that you want to use food to help, take a second to locate on the outline where you feel the emotion. It might be in more than one place. You can map your emotions like this over time and see if there are any patterns or precipitating events, such as a fight with your partner.

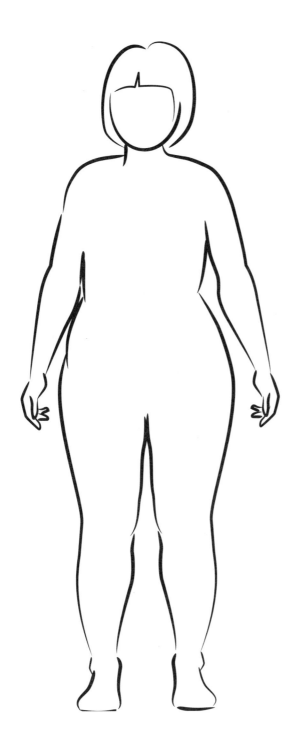

FILLING UP YOUR EMOTIONAL HUNGER

Once you've identified what it is you're feeling, it's time to take action and consider how to meet those emotional needs. Let's be clear, though: eating a piece of cake after a shitty day is *totally* OK, but it might not be giving us everything we need in that moment. Remember the ways in which it might have been helpful for you or served a purpose; the goal here is not to go cold turkey on emotional eating but to build up your emotional coping toolkit so that food isn't your only option.

I like to think of physical hunger being filled by food going into your stomach. Physical hunger can only be met by regular meals and snacks. Once you've had enough to eat, your physical hunger is satisfied. Emotional hunger can't be met with just food. In order to determine how to meet our emotional needs, we have to consider all the things that fill our hearts.

Using the outlines opposite, write out the things that fill your stomach and satisfy your physical hunger, versus the things that fill your heart and satisfy your emotional hunger.

Ideas for things that can satisfy physical hunger:

* regular meals and snacks

* eating a wide range and variety of foods

* being flexible in my approach to eating

* no food rules!

* no restrictions!

Ideas for things that can satisfy our emotional hunger:

Naps	Buying yourself flowers	Faith	Calling a friend	Setting boundaries and saying 'no'	Listening to podcasts	Baking/cooking	Yoga
Being valued in your community	Letting your hair down	Going to museums	Talking to a loved one	Crying	Getting hugs and physical touch	Finding community	Listening to music
Creative writing	Rest	Getting a manicure	Spirituality	Poetry	Dancing	Having fulfilling work	Embodiment
Checking in with family	Journaling	Going dancing with your buddies	Learning new things	Being in nature	Regular friend dates	Going to therapy	
Travel	Making art	Enough sleep	Reading books	Spending time with animals	Meditation	Spending time with special people in your life	

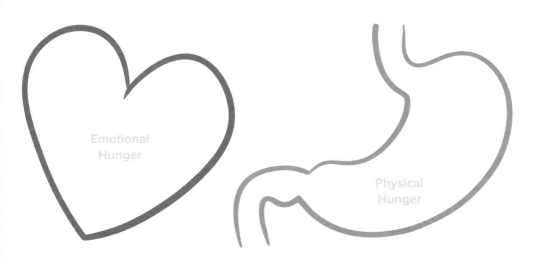

Emotional Hunger

Physical Hunger

EXPANDING YOUR TOOLKIT

In the rest of this chapter, we're going to focus on more skills we can add to our Intuitive Eating Toolkit (from Chapter 1). As with all the tools and skills in the book, play around with them and find what works for you. Different tools will resonate with different people at different times, so if you don't instantly connect with something, don't write it off. Maybe come back to it when you're in a different headspace, and see if it resonates differently.

Five strategies for everyday self-care

Adapted from Susan Abers, eatingmindfully.com

I was working with a client once who was struggling with intense work stress from working in a high-pressure office environment. She felt like food was her only coping mechanism, and alongside working on self-compassion for using food as a coping mechanism, we agreed that it would be a good idea to build some other tools into her toolkit. I asked her what she liked to do to de-stress, and she said she enjoyed going for a swim. Now, don't get me wrong, swimming can be really meditative, and a nice escape from phones and email. But how practical is it, in the middle of the work day, or when you have a screaming toddler, to get your swimming stuff together, get yourself to the pool, change into your swimsuit, have a swim, get out of the pool, shower, put your clothes back on, dry your hair, redo your make-up, and get back to the office or the screaming toddler? Right, not so easy.

That's why in clinic we get clients to put together their 'list of 5s'. That is:

* 5 lists

* of 5 things

* you can do for 5 minutes

These should be low-key self-care strategies that you can engage in fully if you're feeling overwhelmed with anxiety or worry, or are ruminating on a problem, or just feel really stuck in your head. When you're in this headspace, it can be hard to think of ways to engage your mind differently, so having this list somewhere easy to see can be super helpful; you can draw it out and stick it on the fridge, snap a pic, or keep it as a note on your phone.

Critically, these strategies should be easy, convenient, accessible anywhere/anytime, free (or cheap). Going to get your nails done is great – but it doesn't fit these criteria. Whereas painting your nails at home might be a good distraction for 5 minutes!

You'll probably want to make multiple lists – one for home, one for work, one for visiting family, and so on – feel free to make as many as you need for different scenarios.

Complete your list of everyday self-care:

	5 people to call/ text when you feel down or upset, or need to vent	5 ways to relax	5 places you can go to calm down	5 things you can say to yourself	5 activities to distract yourself
1					
2					
3					
4					
5					

HOW TO JUST EAT IT

Because I know people find it tough to fill this out, here are some ideas of the types of things that could go in here:

5 people: friend, sibling, parent, colleague, partner – sometimes there aren't always 5 people who are going to 'get it', but is there someone you could text who you know will send you a funny meme, tell a joke, or otherwise cheer you up?

5 ways to relax: practise deep breathing (I love the 'breathe bubble' in the *Calm* app, which you can set a 5-minute timer for). Mindfully make a herbal tea and notice the steam from the water, the colour changing as the bag infuses, the aroma and the warmth of the mug, and, of course, the taste when you eventually drink it. Stretch; run your hands under cool water; grab a stress ball or some Play-Doh (you can get tiny little pots you can carry in your bag with you).

5 places you can go: this will depend on where you are, but try and think on a micro level, rather than a macro one. For instance, at home it might be: a comfy chair, your bed, or grounding yourself quite literally by lying on the floor (throw down a yoga mat if you haven't vacuumed in a while). At work it might be: a prayer, meditation, or meeting room, stepping outside to a bench, going to another floor to see a colleague.

5 things you can say to yourself: this can feel contrived if you aren't used to using mantras or affirmation, so find something that clicks for you. A favourite of mine comes from a client I worked with who used to say 'chuck it in the fuck-it bucket'. It could also be 'this is really shit right now, but I am strong enough to get through it'. Or it could be something simple like 'you're OK, you've got this'. If you get stuck, a quick search on Google, Pinterest, or Instagram can turn up some good stuff.

5 activities: thinking of little things to do for 5 minutes can be hard, so here are some that seem to resonate with my clients: watching cute puppy or kitten videos on YouTube, scrolling through a 'collection' on Instagram (you could make a collection for animals, travel, intuitive eating or body compassion quotes – whatever makes you feel good!), doing a puzzle/playing a game on your phone, sketching or doodling, playing with a pet.

Self-compassion

Self-compassion is another really neat tool for our toolkit; research is showing that self-compassion is associated with lower levels of anxiety and depression, less disordered eating, and higher body satisfaction, optimism, motivation, and life satisfaction. And sure, it can sound intuitive and simple, but when shit hits the fan, we can often really struggle to do it in real time. That's why I think it's helpful to look at self-compassion as a practice – something we can do in a sequential, step-by-step way until it becomes more natural.

According to researcher and Professor of Psychology at the University of Texas Austin, Kristin Neff, there are three domains of self-compassion:[3-4]

Self-kindness: This refers to our ability to treat ourselves gently and kindly, as we might do a friend. For many of us, when things are tough, we have a tendency to internalize the blame and talk ourselves down. Dieting is a perfect example of this: think back to a time when you've been on a diet or pseudo-diet and then fallen off the wagon; how have you responded? Did you ruminate on all the things you could or should have done better, like 'I should have meal-prepped better' or 'I could have said no to dessert at dinner last night'? This can lead to feelings of stress and frustration. Or did you treat yourself more like a friend would and cut yourself some slack: 'Diets are miserable, and don't work, and you're great just the way you are.' In other words, do you build yourself up, comfort and soothe yourself, or tear yourself down and trash-talk yourself? Putting ourselves down undermines our ability to self-soothe and comfort ourselves when we're in pain and in need of care.

Common humanity: The second tenet of self-compassion has to do with our shared experience with other people. To put it into terms relevant to this book, everyone has weird shit going on with food. OK, maybe not everyone, but it's certainly a lot of people. However, because we don't really talk about our stuff, we rarely consider that other people are also struggling with their relationship to food, exercise, or body image. As Neff puts it: 'All humans are flawed works-in-progress; everyone fails, makes mistakes, and engages in dysfunctional behaviour. All of us reach for things we cannot have, and have to remain in the presence of difficult experiences that we desperately want to avoid.' When we take a myopic view, we get it in our heads that everyone else is nailing it: diets, exercise, relationships, parenting, career, spirituality, creativity, life in general. But literally no one has all their shit together, at least not all of the time. Remind yourself that everyone has ups and downs, and that the intuitive eating process is no different. I don't mean to freak you out by saying that, but to reassure you that you're not fucking it up. Self-compassion can help us feel less isolated when we are in pain, by recognizing our common humanity and shared experiences. We're all in this together.

Mindful awareness: Mindfulness speaks to our ability to witness emotions, thoughts, and sensations without judgement, avoidance, or repression. Why is this important in the context of self-compassion? Well, you need to be able to first of all recognize that you are suffering or in pain in order to give yourself compassion. An example I see of this is of people who use food to 'numb out'. They use food to push down uncomfortable emotions. Sometimes this is an important coping mechanism, but if viewed without mindful self-compassion, we might miss the fact that emotional eating may be a symptom that something else is going on for us. Bringing a gentle awareness allows us to bear witness to our experience, even when it's uncomfortable. Mindfulness also prevents us from over-identifying with a particular feeling or emotion to the point that we can no longer differentiate ourselves from our thoughts. 'That kinda sucks' becomes 'I suck'; 'that was disappointing' becomes 'I'm a disappointment'. Mindfulness allows us to examine our thoughts as simply that – thoughts. Not facts. That in turn can put a little distance between you and your thoughts so you don't over-identify with them.

SELF-COMPASSION PRACTICES

Let's step through each of these components with a self-compassion practice.

MINDFUL AWARENESS

The first step is to mindfully acknowledge that we're experiencing a tough or challenging situation or emotion. Mindful awareness of our experience allows us to intercept with some love and kindness directed towards ourselves, therefore breaking the usual loop of negative self-talk.

Pick one of the following:

* Things are really tough for me right now.

* This sucks.

* This is a moment of suffering.

* I'm having a tough time.

* I'm really struggling today.

* ....

COMMON HUMANITY

The second step is to recognize that suffering is a universal experience and that you're not alone in feeling this way. The flavour of suffering is different from person to person, but we're all dealing with something difficult. This can help us recognize that we'd offer other people compassion if they were experiencing the same feelings as we are now; sometimes we find it easier to send compassion to others, but can we also direct it back towards ourselves?

Pick one of the following:

* I'm not alone in feeling this way.

* Other people feel this way – and we all matter.

* I'm having a human experience – other people feel this way too.

* I've felt this way before and have survived.

* ....

SELF-KINDNESS

The last step is to offer ourselves some loving kindness. This can be the hardest step, so take some time to think about what you might say to yourself. If words don't resonate, then can you imagine giving yourself a hug, or wrapping yourself in a blanket of kindness?
Pick one of the following:

* May I be well, may we all be well.

* I'm doing the best I can and it's enough.

* I am kind and strong.

* May I be happy, may I be safe, may I be at peace.

* ....

Gratitude

The last tool we can add to the toolkit is gratitude. Gratitude is linked with life satisfaction, optimism, hope, positive disposition, empathy, and forgiveness. A regular gratitude practice may also help reduce body dissatisfaction and disordered eating symptoms. Sounds great, right? But how does it work practically? There's no point in just reeling off a bunch of things you're grateful for, just for the sake of it. A key part of keeping a gratitude journal is actually channelling a sense of gratitude while you're writing. For instance, think about how you feel when you see your favourite person, or hear your favourite song. You might have a warm, tingly feeling, or a sense of calm and peace – fostering these feelings while you're writing in your journal is part of the process.

In your journal, take five minutes to list out five things you're grateful for, focusing on the feelings that the item conjures up. A sense of warmth, calm, reassurance, peacefulness, loving kindness, hopefulness, fulfilment, or joy. The benefits of a gratitude practice are cumulative, so try and set aside five minutes a day to run through your gratitude list – even if you don't have a chance to write it down.

✚ Can you recognize the purpose and function behind your emotional eating?

✚ Are you able to approach it with a sense of kindness and curiosity, or are you still being tough on yourself?

✚ Are there any tools from this section that you can add to your toolkit? Go back to Chapter 1 and write them in.

✚ If you look back, have you noticed any fairy lights coming on?

Listen to the corresponding podcast episode Don't Salt My Game – How to Just Eat It: Chapter 6

CHAPTER 6

LETTING GO OF FOOD RULES

This section is appropriate for people in eating disorder recovery, although it might be helpful to work through the activities alongside your treatment team to get the most out of it. This is an integral part of challenging the eating disorder voice, but it's important to make sure you're at a point in your recovery where you're ready to do so.

Look, I get it. The idea of giving yourself full, unconditional permission to eat whatever you feel like eating can feel scary and overwhelming. But it's a critical step in making peace with and healing our relationship with food. To help us understand this a bit better, I want to use a metaphor developed by therapist Deb Burgard, called 'Dietland to Doughnutland'. What happens when we pull a pendulum all the way to one side? It picks up momentum and swings all the way to the other side, right? And unless we intervene, it keeps bouncing back and forth from side to side. Going on a diet is like pulling the pendulum all the way to one side – Deb calls this dietland. When we let go of the pendulum, it immediately swings all the way to the other side: doughnutland. The harder we pull into dietland, the harder and faster we swing into doughnutland. But what happens when we leave a pendulum alone and just let it be? It finds a point between these two extremes where it sits, effortlessly. Sure, it may oscillate a little back and forth, but there are no longer these vicious swings from dietland to doughnutland. This settling point is where I conceptualize intuitive eating: a point where you're not in a binge–restrict cycle. You feel pretty neutral about foods and can eat in a varied, balanced, and flexible way without feeling restricted or deprived.

Does the dietland to doughnutland pendulum analogy resonate with your own experiences? Can you notice what happens when you pull the pendulum to dietland? Do you feel the draw to swing back to doughnutland?

On the diagram below, note where you fall currently on the pendulum.

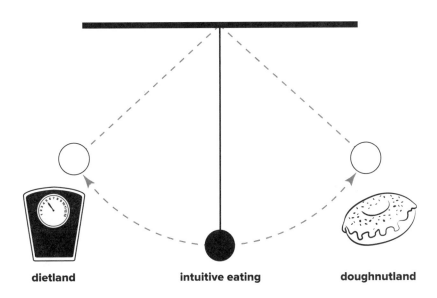

dietland   **intuitive eating**   **doughnutland**

Food and diet rules keep us trapped in this persistent swinging from one extreme to another; that's why intuitive eating invites us to *break the rules* and give ourselves *unconditional permission to eat*.

I get that this sounds weird coming from a nutrition professional, so let's break it down a little because it's not as weird as it sounds. Unlike what the gym bros on Instagram have to say, giving ourselves unconditional permission to eat does not mean 'fuck it, eat whatever you want whenever you want'. What it actually refers to is making peace with foods that we have restricted and deprived ourselves of; foods that fill us up and satisfy us emotionally and physically. The natural response to this sense of scarcity is to eat past comfortable fullness (or perhaps even binge) on foods that we have told ourselves we 'can't' or 'shouldn't' have. Even if we are physically eating these so-called 'bad' foods, the act of psychologically ring-fencing a food or food group can trigger a sense of deprivation and scarcity which heightens our desire for the thing we can't have. This is commonly known as the forbidden fruit effect – think about what happens if you tell a toddler they can't play with the iPad. Are they all 'yeah, OK, cool' and get right back to their stickers? *Nope*. Full-on meltdown ensues. We may not externally melt down when we can't have the foods we love, but we sure as shit have a little internal food FOMO freak-out. It can create a sense of urgency, intensity, and deep desire for the thing you can't have, the forbidden fruit. But of course you can have that food if you really want it, and if you violate the terms of this cognitive boundary you have placed around food, you might end up triggering the *fuck-it effect*. You know what I mean. 'Well, I've had a cookie now, fuck it, might as well have ten.' In other words, a sense of deprivation not only makes us feel obsessed and preoccupied with food, but it can set us up to feel out of control; when we finally do eat a particular food, it can result in eating past the point of comfortable fullness, eating in the absence of hunger, or binge eating.

This can reinforce the idea that we have no willpower and can't be trusted around food – we might even say we're 'addicted' to food. Instead, by giving ourselves unconditional permission to eat all foods (yes, even carbs and sugar!) we begin to dismantle the scarcity mindset that can make us feel weird around food in the first place.

 Another helpful way to think about what's going on here is based on a metaphor that Eliza on my team came up with (thanks E!).

I want you to hold your breath for as long as you can possibly stand it. Start counting in your mind – 1, 2, 3, and so on. Keep going until you can't go any longer.

Don't just read this, I want you to actually do it.

OK, before you pass out – take a deep breath in. Give yourself a few moments to let your breathing return to normal.

Notice how, when you deprived yourself of oxygen for a period of time, you didn't immediately go back to regular breathing – you probably took a huge deep breath that filled your lungs to the point that they felt like they might pop. Then you probably needed at least a few long, deep breaths, or perhaps you got the hiccups! It takes some time to readjust back to having adequate oxygen and being able to breathe whenever and however we want. The same thing is true for food – if we restrict and deprive ourselves of foods that we love and enjoy, then our bodies are going to try hard to make up for it – similarly to how our bodies try to make up for not having enough oxygen. Although it only takes a few moments to catch our breath, it can take time for our bodies to feel like they're no longer deprived of previously off-limits foods. Look back at page 117 – our bodies need to learn to trust us as much as we need to learn to trust our bodies.

HABITUATION

As long as we keep foods up on a pedestal and never allow ourselves to eat them, the novelty never wears off; we never habituate to them. In other words, we never learn how to be around those foods without them causing us stress or us feeling out of control around them. Habituation explains what happens when we are consistently exposed to a stimulus, over and over, so that it loses its power to affect us. For example, when I first moved to London, I struggled to sleep because of the noise from sirens – now I barely notice them. It's also why parents 'rotate' kids' toys; after a while kids get bored of a toy, but put it in the cupboard until they forget about it, and it's like a whole new toy again.

The same thing is true of food. In a classic experiment, women were given macaroni and cheese every day for a week. Living the dream, right? At the beginning of the week they were all like 'woohoo, mac and cheese!', but by the end of the week, they were kind of over it, essentially getting a bit bored of the macaroni.[1] Similar effects have been shown with a wide variety of foods – everything from milk and cheese and crackers to pizza and burgers.[2, 3]

Scientists believe that the time it takes to habituate to a food is less when the food shares similar characteristics (for instance, the same flavour and brand of ice cream), which is why I'm going to ask you to get really specific when we reintroduce foods from your shit list – you know that place where all 'bad' foods live in your mind? Yeah, that's your shit list.

We need to remember, though, that the point of giving yourself unconditional permission to eat all foods isn't to get so burnt out on a food that you never want to eat it again; I don't want you to eat so much pizza or ice cream or bagels that you make yourself sick and swear off them for good, because that would result in restriction and deprivation, which would be self-defeating. You'd be back at square one. The point in food habituation is to really bring those foods down off that pedestal so they no longer have the same emotional pull. You don't have to eat them with such an urgency or intensity, and you can have them when you really want them, as opposed to when you feel compelled or drawn to them.

In this section, we'll break down that cognitive boundary around good and bad foods and replace it with food neutrality. We'll decimate food rules and restrictions and learn to eat according to what our body wants and needs and what makes us feel good! We'll kick the scarcity mindset in the face so we can make food choices from a place of security and stability, without the threat of future deprivation, to nourish our bodies and souls! Getting back to a place where you are no longer restricting foods that you crave and giving yourself full, unconditional permission to eat is a process and can take some time.

EXAMINING YOUR FOOD RULES

 In your journal write a list of the rules you have around what, when, or how much you eat. You may not even be aware of all of your food rules initially – many will be subconscious – so pay attention to what crops up when you go out to dinner, or if you have multiple portions of carbs in the same day. Whatever it is, write it down, and then answer the following questions.

* How do these rules help facilitate joy and pleasure around eating?

* How do these rules allow me flexibility in my eating?

* How do these rules give me the space to discover the foods I really enjoy and want to eat?

* How are these rules helping or holding me back from trusting my own ability to regulate the amount of food that's comfortable and satisfying for me?

* How do these rules stop me from paying attention to my own hunger and fullness signals?

* How do these rules help me become an intuitive eater?

What's on your shit list?

Our shit lists are the running lists of 'bad' foods we create in our minds. They tend to be a weird mixture of remnants of diets past, food that wellness culture deems inedible (like gluten), some stuff that was on our parents' shit list, plus some stuff you read in a magazine. This list that we carry around in our minds serves to reinforce scarcity and feelings of deprivation and restriction – even if the list itself is subconscious. That's why I think it's really helpful to write it all down. Some things I see commonly on shit lists include:

* 'Processed' foods

* Sweet foods like chocolate, ice cream, and pastries

* Takeaways – pizza, Chinese food, fish and chips

* Starchy foods like bread, potatoes, pasta, rice, crisps

* Foods that are higher in fat, even if they're 'healthier' foods like avocado or nuts

In your journal, write out your shit list. You could also make a visual representation of your shit list using your food icons (see appendix page 313). You could use Blu Tack to stick them up on the wall. The foods towards the top tend to be the ones you feel worst about eating (perhaps even binge foods) or maybe restrict completely. Whereas the ones lower down you might feel mild pangs of guilt about for a little while after eating but are more comfortable with.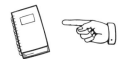

+ Are you surprised by the number of foods on your list?

+ What is the result of restricting or depriving yourself of these foods?

+ How does having this list interfere with your ability to eat intuitively?

+ How can you cultivate food neutrality towards these foods?

+ Can you stop thinking of them in terms of good/bad, healthy/ unhealthy, etc?

Notice that you have created a food hierarchy and how establishing this cognitive boundary around food might actually contribute to heightened cravings and feelings of loss of control around those foods. We can begin to contemplate what it might be like if we were to actually give ourselves permission to eat those foods. We might fear that we will swing all the way into doughnutland, and maybe we will for a while, but how about in the long term? If we stop pulling the pendulum so hard, does it help us find a natural settling point?

FOOD NEUTRALITY

A great stepping stone towards giving yourself unconditional permission to eat is practising what I like to call food neutrality. Basically, it means getting over all our judgey stuff about food and looking at food as something neutral, from a moral perspective. Food does not imbue us with morality; we are not virtuous for eating kale and sinners for eating cake.

Step 1 – Check yourself before you wreck yourself

Check yourself: how are you talking to yourself and others about food? A simple step we can begin to implement almost immediately is neutralizing our language and becoming non-judgey about how we label foods. Let's take a look at the language we use around food.

How many of the following words do you use to describe foods?

good	clean	protein*
bad	dirty	fat*
naughty	real	carb*
guilt-free	fake	heavy
light	junk food	indulgent
all natural	healthy	guilty pleasure
processed	unhealthy	sin foods
refined	contains 'chemicals'	x points/calories/macros
contains 'nasties'	treat	

* I tend to avoid using nutrient-based names of foods because they are often loaded with judgement – for example, protein is seen as the wonder nutrient whereas carbs get a bad rap. We need them both: neither is better than the other, they just fulfil different functions in the body. And good luck pooping without carbs

Try to catch yourself when you notice you are using these terms to describe food – there is a whole neutral vocabulary we can use to describe food that is a lot less judgemental and fosters a kinder relationship with food. When it comes to describing foods or food groups, instead of calling them 'good' or 'bad', let's try using their actual names. So a salad, pastry, burrito, cheese. For food groups, we can call them dairy, vegetables, meat, fish, bread/pasta/grains, fruit, sweets, nuts, etc. Here are some more neutral words you can use to describe food:

breakfast	elevenses	satisfying
lunch	afters	delicious
dinner	pudding	tasty
brunch	supper	mouth-watering
snack	sweet	bland
dessert	savoury	creamy
starter	wholesome	hearty
entrée	refreshing	
main course	comforting	

Step 2 – Examine your belief in the concept of a 'perfect' diet

Diet culture has us believe that there are such things as 'good' foods and 'bad' foods. That there are 'good' and 'bad' diets. That we can 'optimize' our diet to achieve 'perfect' health. All of this is bullshit. Yes, food can play a role in supporting overall health, but it's not the be-all and end-all. This rhetoric can be so damaging because it essentially says you are to blame if your health goes to shit. It's placing individual responsibility on a complex social issue.

What's also really problematic is the moralism we project onto foods – if someone eats a so-called 'good' food, we ascribe that person a higher moral value; we assume they are pure and wholesome. Likewise 'bad' food, 'bad' people. At least this is the subtext.

> Reflect for a moment on the type of person you associate with eating at McDonald's, or the type of person who loads up their shopping trolley with convenience foods. What stories do you tell yourself about that person, their health, their character? Do you feel a sense of moral superiority when you're eating an organic kale salad?

My intention is not to make you feel bad – I've been that person who scans someone's shopping basket, looking for clues to judge them by (in fact, I think it was baked into my nutrition training). What I want to highlight here is that we – often unconsciously – judge people based on their food choices. Including ourselves. Try and notice if you do this – remember that we don't know about the hundreds of different factors that go into someone else's food choices, and how much or little control they may have over them.

Using the food icons (see appendix, page 313) from your shit list, can you symbolically place them all on an even playing field by laying them out into one long line? I love doing this in clinic with clients because it ends up looking like the pages of *The Very Hungry Caterpillar* (yeah, now you have the image!).

Step 3 – Don't think of nutrition in black and white terms

We can be very all or nothing when it comes to food and nutrition. Thinking that a handful of chips cancels out the essential nutrients in fish and peas. Nutrition is not a zero-sum game, but we tend to dichotomize our eating as 'good' or 'bad', 'healthy' or 'unhealthy'.

Nutrition professionals have a lot to answer for here too – we often use labels like 'good' fats and 'good' carbs. Or 'bad' fats and 'bad' carbs. This misses so much context and nuance. For instance, for a diabetic or an athlete who needs a quick source of glucose a bowl of quinoa isn't going to cut it, even if we label it as a 'good' carb. Likewise, dairy can be high in the 'bad' saturated fats, but it's also a really important source of protein, calcium, and iodine. See, not so simple – food is a complicated mixture of different chemical components. It's impossible to categorize them as good or bad, despite how hard we try.

Instead of looking at the minutiae of detail in an individual food, what if we could take a step back and notice patterns of eating over time? Not with judgement or criticism, but with, you guessed it, curiosity? How do I feel when I don't eat many vegetables? Do I feel fuller and more satisfied after I've had a balanced plate? Do I notice my cravings intensifying when I don't allow myself to regularly eat enjoyable foods?

Step 4 – Look at the bigger picture of health

Working with clients, I've noticed that we tend to overplay the role that nutrition has in our overall health and well-being. That's not to say that nutrition isn't meaningful and important in terms of keeping us well, but that we over-hype it in relation to other contributors to our health.

I want you to imagine that the following is a pie chart of 'health' – health means different things to different people, but I want you to think about what it means to you. Divide your pie up into all the different slices that contribute to giving you a sense of health and well-being in their relative proportions (e.g. 25 per cent nutrition, 25 per cent exercise, etc)

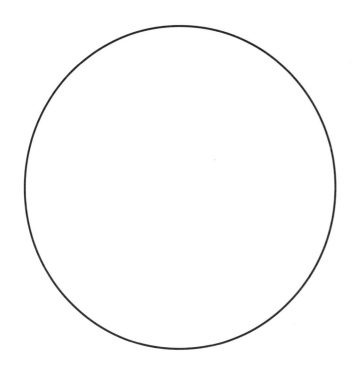

Now take a look at the following chart, which shows the relative contributing factors that make us healthy at a population level. Granted, comparing this to your individual answers is tricky, but what I want you to take away from this is that health is more than the sum of our individual behaviours. Much more than if we're eating 5-a-day, or what the number on the scales says. Health falls along a socio-economic gradient – if we are relatively privileged, we will automatically, without even trying, live longer, healthier lives, than those living in, chronic poverty or deprivation.[4]

For a more in-depth discussion of this topic, listen to episode 76 of my podcast Don't Salt My Game – When Public Health Totally Misses the Point with Dr Oli Williams

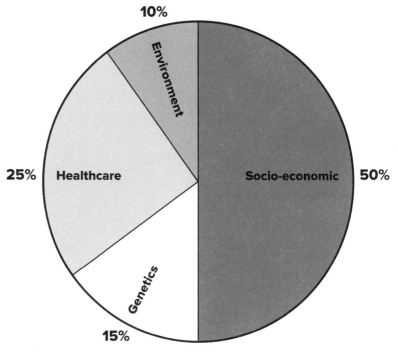

The Social Determinants of Health (income, housing, unemployment, education etc.) account for 50% of health status

Canadian Institute of Advanced Research, Health Canada, Population and Public Health Branch. AB/NWT 2002

✛ What has the biggest influence over our health and well-being?

✛ What are some of the structural and social barriers to health equality?

✛ If we were all to eat the same, would we have the same health outcomes or weight?

Step 5 – Fuck food guilt

An important step in practising food neutrality is rejecting food guilt, but that's perhaps harder to do when all we hear are messages about 'guilty pleasures', 'being naughty', and 'bad food'. It's hard not to internalize these messages, which manifest as a mixture of sadness and frustration directed back at ourselves. Guilt and shame can follow us around for days after a perceived food transgression. But who decided you should feel guilty about enjoying foods? Who told you that you were bad for nourishing your soul with foods that satisfy you? That's some grade A, puritanical, patriarchal, fat-phobic, diet culture BS. None of us were born with food rules, but years and years of diets (even the ones masquerading as 'lifestyles'), fashion magazines, and thin-ideal idolization erode our trust in our body's cues and our innate ability to feed ourselves. Diet culture teaches us that we cannot be trusted around delicious foods. It teaches that you need to have strategies in place to deal with all the food because YOU CANNOT BE TRUSTED.

Well, guess what? You are a grown adult who gets to eat whatever you like, whenever you like, and enjoy the crap out of it! If feelings of guilt, shame, or anxiety creep in, remind yourself those are not *your* feelings, they were given to you by a culture that preys on your insecurities and vulnerabilities. But you are done with diet culture now, and you are not going to let it walk all over you. Not today. Not next week or next month. Not ever. Eating is a fundamental requirement for life. You would not feel guilty about breathing or sleeping. You should never, ever feel bad about nourishing your body and soul with satisfying and delicious foods that help keep body and mind happy. YOU ARE DONE WITH FOOD GUILT because you deserve to enjoy all the pleasure that food has to offer, there is no space left for feeling guilty, and you will not let diet culture dull your sparkle.

It's natural that you will have some concerns about moving through the IE process, and at some point you may feel as though food consumes your every waking second, and 'AAAARRRGGGHHH, this was supposed to help me think less about food, not more!' Chill. The ultimate goal in IE is to think less about food, but in the early stages of IE it's totally normal for there to be a period where we are hyper-focused on food choices. Be curious about it. It doesn't mean you're screwing it up. It's part of the process. Speaking of which, if you feel like you're down with the food neutrality stuff, let's look at a stepped approach to reintroducing off-limits or forbidden foods from your shit list.

PUTTING UNCONDITIONAL PERMISSION INTO PRACTICE

This activity helps facilitate the habituation process, with a little bit of structure so you don't feel so overwhelmed or out of control – adding in previously forbidden foods should be a positive experience, not one that stresses you out! However, if you do find yourself feeling overwhelmed, check in with your toolkit and remind yourself of what you might need so you can have a good experience with this food. I'll walk you through the steps, and then there's a planning tool you can use to actually put unconditional permission to eat into practice.

Step 1 – Select your shit list food

Flip back to page 184 and find your shit list; pick one food that you would like to have a better relationship with. Depending on your confidence level, you might want to pick something in the middle of the list, which pushes you outside your comfort zone but doesn't totally freak you out. If you're feeling trepidation, pick something lower down that's only just outside your comfort zone.

Step 2 – Get specific

Once you've chosen your food, decide which brand and flavour you want to work towards giving yourself unconditional permission to eat. Say, for instance, it's ice cream, you might want to start with Ben & Jerry's Phish Food. Then you can go to Cookie Dough flavour or whichever other flavour you want to get cosy with. Being specific is important; if you just pick chocolate, well, there are so many different brands and flavours that it will take longer to habituate. Keeping it specific can also feel a bit less frightening and help you build confidence.

Step 3 – Make a plan

Decide when and where you're going to have the food, using the questions below to guide you. You could start by keeping smaller amounts in the house, and then work towards keeping your cupboards stocked.

* Are you going to have it at home, or out (say at your favourite restaurant)?

* Do you need to try this alone, or will you get some support from a caring friend or partner?

* How many times over the next week are you going to attempt this food? (Note that once a week is not enough for habituation; research suggests it should ideally be four or five times per week.)

* Are you going to have it as part of a meal or snack, on its own, or mix it up?

 Use the following prompts to make a plan; you can write these out in your journal as you may want to attempt it with more than one food:

Food from shit list I want to have a better relationship with:

Brand:

Flavour:

Any other details (snack pack, family size, etc):

Where am I going to have this food?

Will I have it as part of a meal/snack?

What time of day will I have it?

Who will be there when I have it?

Step 4 – Get your head straight

Check in with yourself and make sure you're in the right headspace for this. Are you approaching it with the mentality that you're going to binge and 'overeat' it (which runs the risk of becoming a self-fulfilling prophecy), or can you approach it with mindful, non-judgemental awareness? Also pay attention to whether or not you're stressed, over-hungry or tired, as these can all influence how much you eat. If you're experiencing any of these things and feel there's a danger you will have a negative experience with the food, maybe come back to it later when you're rested and feeling good.

Step 5 – Goldilocks that shit

Have the food as per your plan and then start asking questions. Goldilocks that shit: how much is too little, too much, just right for you to leave you feeling content, but not so stuffed you feel sick, or so restricted you feel deprived? Or maybe you don't actually want ice cream but cheese on toast or a doughnut? How did it go? How did the food taste? As good as you expected, or was it slightly disappointing? Was the experiment pleasant, unpleasant, or neutral? Did you eat more or less than you expected?

There's no right or wrong answer. You're just gathering information. The first few times you try this, you might eat a lot of the food, more than is comfortable; remember that's totally normal when you're trying to reverse the deprivation mindset. Notice if on subsequent eating experiences the amount of food you eat goes up or down. What often happens is that people require smaller amounts of the food to feel satisfied; this can take different lengths of time for different people, so it's impossible to say how many times you need to repeat this activity before you start to feel like you're giving yourself unconditional permission. Remember what we talked about at the very beginning? Patience!

Using the following template, you can 'Goldilocks' the food you want to have a better relationship with (as decided in step 3). I typically recommend giving yourself a week of intentionally including this food as part of a meal or snack (although you may need more or less time, depending on how challenging the food feels). Complete this in your journal so you can repeat it for other foods.

DAY	1	2
How am I feeling beforehand? If I am relaxed or stressed, is this related to the food or is there something else going on for me? (work, relationships, etc)		
Physical hunger cues		
Emotional cues		
When I last ate		
What do I need right now to feel more comfortable with this practice? (taking some deep breaths, getting fresh air, eating with someone)		
How did the food taste? (delicious, satisfying, disappointing, hit the spot, not what I was craving, unsatisfying)		
How did I feel afterwards? (content, comfortably full, uncomfortably full, satisfied)		
How much did it take me to feel content and satisfied?		
What's my self-talk like? Am I judging myself for how much or the type of food eaten?		

Rate your level of comfort with this food at the start of the week:
/ **10**

Rate your level of comfort with this food at the end of the week:
/ **10**

3	4	5	6	7

> **Unconditional permission to eat activity**
>
> + Has this activity changed your perceptions or beliefs about this food?
>
> + Were your assumptions about this food true? Was it as daunting as you thought it would be?
>
> + Did you notice your comfort level or confidence with this food increase over time?
>
> + If you had to put this food back on your shit list, would it still be in the same position as it was before?

Step 6 – Rinse and repeat

Repeat the experiment until you begin to experience unconditional permission to eat that food. There's no hard and fast test for this, but here are some things to look out for:

* I don't feel guilt, shame, or anxiety about this food any more.

* I don't feel a super intense desire for this food any more – I could take it or leave it.

* I could have this food in the house and not feel as though I would demolish it in one sitting.

* I don't need to engage in any compensatory behaviours to 'earn' this food.

* I don't think this food is good or bad, healthy or unhealthy, it's just food.

Don't judge how many times or how much of the food you need to eat in order to feel comfortable with it. If you've been restricting for a long time and are deep in a deprivation mindset then it may take longer; this can be frustrating, so remember to approach it with a sense of curiosity, like an experiment. You don't know what the results will be until you've finished the experiment and it may or may not prove your hypothesis.

Giving yourself unconditional permission to eat expands your comfort zone, so once you've given yourself unconditional permission to eat one food, it's time to try the next one on your shit list. This time try going a step higher on the list, gently nudging yourself outside the new comfort zone. You'll probably only need to do this with a handful of foods before you start to internalize unconditional permission for all foods. You'll be flexing that intuitive eating muscle, and the more you do that, the less you'll need to be so methodical in your approach to eating; you'll be able to trust that you can eat all foods without conditions, without rules, or without having to justify it to yourself or anyone else.

+ How does it feel giving yourself unconditional permission to eat any foods you like?

+ Do you still notice yourself judging food choices, or are you becoming more neutral about them?

+ Are you feeling any more confident eating shit list foods? If not, what would help increase your confidence?

+ Reflect on whether or not any more fairy lights have come on for you!

+ Are there any tools from this section that you can add to your toolkit? Go back to Chapter 1 and write them in).

Listen to the corresponding podcast episode Don't Salt My Game – How to Just Eat It: Chapter 7

CHAPTER 7

NEUTRALIZING THE INNER FOOD CRITIC

For those with an eating disorder, learning how to reframe unhelpful thoughts around food can help you make choices that align with recovery rather than with the eating disorder voice. It can be hard to differentiate your authentic voice from the eating disorder voice at first, so make sure you have the appropriate support to help you do this.

We're not born knowing how to criticize food – put a selection of foods in front of a baby who is learning how to eat and they won't do a quick equation to figure out how many grams of protein, fat, and carbs are in that food. They don't care about 'refined sugar' or gluten or antioxidants. They eat, they play with food, they make a huge mess, and most importantly they connect with food using their senses. It's not until they're much older that they start to learn the rules of diet culture: it might start in school with healthy eating lessons, or be learned via their parents' dieting rules, but ultimately they learn these rules from diet and wellness cultures that install morality into food choices. Unlike the baby who uses their instinct to explore food and learn their own food preferences (through natural contingency – see the Introduction, page 29), food rules are installed in us like an annoying update on your phone that you didn't want and that slows everything down. These food rules collude with our natural tendency to be our own harshest judge; I call this the *inner food critic*. In this section we're going to begin to notice how we talk to ourselves about food; this awareness is fundamental to beginning to change our self-talk and can help us give ourselves unconditional permission to eat, as well as to be kinder to ourselves overall.

HOW DO YOU TALK TO YOURSELF ABOUT FOOD?

A common place people get tripped up when giving themselves unconditional permission to eat is their self-talk. Sure, you might be eating the food, but is permission being undermined by the inner food critic and causing psychological sabotage? We need to better understand how your inner food critic operates. You could note down what your self-talk sounds like around food over the course of a day; we're just bringing some gentle awareness to what that conversation sounds like. This helps us identify the inner food critic so that we can begin to try and reframe or reroute that conversation. It's also important to be aware that these conversations don't take place in a vacuum, so notice what else might be going on for you, following the prompts in the table below. I recommend doing this over a few days so that you can spot patterns and variations over time. Again, the idea here is not to scrutinize your food choices, but to observe your experiences with curiosity and compassion. Keep a note on your phone during the day or write straight in your journal.

Here's an example of what it might look like:

DAY 1

Meal	What I ate	Thoughts around food/body	What else was going on for me? (How was I feeling? Did anything stressful happen? Am I calm?)
Breakfast	Yoghurt, berries, seeds and nuts	Good breakfast, low in carbs, 'on track' for the day	Didn't sleep very well last night but did a spin class this morning
Snack / dessert		Resisting the cake in the office for Sharon's birthday; don't want to end up looking like her	Anxious about my performance review, slumping, need coffee
Lunch	Chicken salad with dressing on the side	Fits my macros	Feeling headachy and having hard time concentrating
Snack / dessert	Rice cake with dark chocolate. Snuck small piece of cake	Feel bloated and guilty	Couldn't stop thinking about the cake so had some chocolate rice cakes instead but then caved in and had a piece but feel disgusting
Dinner	Salmon, broccoli, cauli rice – went back and stole a piece of flatmate's home-made sourdough bread	Have no self-control around carbs, wish flatmate didn't have them in the house to tempt me	Feeling upset by performance review – boss said I lack focus
Snack / dessert	½ jar of peanut butter, several handfuls of granola, tub of yoghurt	Feeling bloated and uncomfortable, worried about gaining weight. Am disgusting for eating this much. Will have to cut back tomorrow and go to back-to-back classes	

As you can see, this individual's inner food critic is harsh and loud and lacking any self-compassion; it also gets angry about things unrelated to food and somehow manages to blame the food.

After completing a few days of checking in with your inner food critic, what did you notice?

✚ Is your inner food critic louder or quieter than you expected?

✚ How would you describe your self-talk around food?

✚ Did you notice any relationship between how you were feeling, what was going on around you, and how you spoke to yourself around food?

Devinia Noel
Intuitive eating counsellor
and CBT therapist
@Thedietboycott

Unhelpful thinking styles – and how to reframe them

For many of us, our inner food critic relies on unhelpful styles of thinking. These types of thoughts can be distressing and can have a negative impact on our relationship with our body and food. The good news is that CBT-based practices can help you develop awareness of your thinking, allowing you to begin to reframe your unhelpful thoughts into more realistic, neutral ones, which in turn helps you become kinder and more compassionate towards yourself. Here are some of the most common types of unhelpful thinking – you might recognize one or more of them.

Black-and-white (all or nothing) thinking Your rationalizing tends to be extreme, without considering any nuance or grey areas in a situation. Things are therefore considered a total success or a complete failure, with no middle ground. You might notice that you're very critical and harsh on yourself if you don't do things 'perfectly'.

For example: after eating a cookie, you may say to yourself 'I've ruined the entire day because I've eaten something sugary' or 'I'm a complete failure because I ate bread for breakfast and dinner. I'm only allowed carbs once a day.'

Mental filter You're unable to consider all the elements of a situation. You tend to filter out the positives and focus on the negatives, without taking into account anything that will make you feel good. You might find you have your mental filter on when you've eaten a food you consider 'bad', without considering the joy eating this food brings.

For example: 'I can't enjoy this chocolate bar because it's full of sugar and fat.'

Catastrophizing You predict that the very worst will happen. When faced with a situation that hasn't gone your way, things get blown out of proportion and feel like an utter disaster. You might find yourself spiralling as you think of all the bad things that could happen. This thinking style is often paired with feelings of anxiety and fear.

For example: I've eaten cake > I'm going to get diabetes > I will be on medication for the rest of my life > I won't be able to live a normal life.

Emotional reasoning You consider your feelings as the objective truth. You find it difficult to distinguish your feelings from the facts, and the way you view situations depends on how you're feeling at the time. If you have critical thoughts about yourself, you might find it harder to see a situation for what it is.

For example: 'I feel guilty that I can't stop bingeing, therefore I must be a bad person.'

Jumping to conclusions You form an opinion about something without having all the facts. There are two main ways people jump to conclusions: by mind reading (when you assume you know what somebody else is thinking about you) and fortune telling (when you predict what will happen in the future based on your feelings).

For example: 'I know they think my food choices are terrible' (mind reading); 'When I visit my family, they're going to be judgemental about my food choices and I'm going to have a horrible time' (fortune telling).

Compare and Despair You compare yourself to other people and tend to see the positives in them, but focus on aspects of yourself you don't like, or view as negative. You tend to disregard your positive qualities in favour of other people, who you assume are in a better situation than you. You might compare your body image and food choices to those of other people.

For example: 'They have so much control around food, yet I'm out of control and I will never be able to have a good relationship with food.'

Labelling You call yourself critical and harsh names based on a particular situation. When something goes wrong, you may see yourself as 'a bad person' or 'stupid'. Your opinion of yourself is focused on negative labels, rather than a holistic view taking in all aspects of the situation.

For example: 'I'm pathetic because I can't stop eating ice cream.'

'Should' and 'must' statements You put yourself under a lot of pressure and feel guilty when you're unable to adhere to the food rules you have set for yourself. You might establish unreasonable rules and put unattainable demands on yourself, which result in feelings of anxiety, low self-esteem and low mood.

For example: 'I must stop eating all my meals by 6pm' or 'I should be able to control myself around food.'

CBT Thought Reframing Exercise

Fill in the following exercise to help reframe your unhelpful thoughts. In case it's useful, an example of a completed exercise can be found below.

1 What is your unhelpful thought? Write down the unhelpful thought that has been triggered by your unhelpful thinking style.

....

What unhelpful thinking style does it represent?

....

2 How does this thought make you feel?

....

How intense is this emotion on a scale of 1–10?

....

3 Consider the evidence for and against your thought.

✖ Evidence for: What evidence suggests that this thought is
   true? Are there any facts that show this thought is accurate?

....

....

✖ Evidence against: What evidence suggests that this thought is
   false? Is there any evidence that can discredit this thought?

....

....

4 Reframe the thought. Look back at your answers to questions
2 and 3. How does this thought make you feel? What does the
evidence for and against suggest? Based on how the thought
makes you feel and the evidence collected, is there another way
for you to look at things – a way that is more compassionate and
neutral? Write down a compassionate and neutral thought.

....

....

....

5. Reflection. How are you feeling now? Have your emotions and thoughts shifted? How can you put your new thoughts into practice on a daily basis? Do you need to work on a particular intuitive eating principle to shift this unhelpful thinking style and thought?

....

....

Here's an example of what this exercise might look like when completed:

1. What is your unhelpful thought?

'I should only eat sugary foods from Friday to Sunday as I can't control myself around them.'

What unhelpful thinking style does it represent?

'Should' and 'must' statements

2. How does this thought make you feel?

'I feel stressed anytime I want to eat anything that isn't fruit or vegetables at the weekend. I feel unhappy and I'm very preoccupied with the foods I've told myself I cannot eat.'

3. Consider the evidence for and against your thought.

Evidence supporting my thought/Facts that show my thought is accurate:

'Health professionals say that it's important to limit my sugar intake for my health. I feel out of control around sugary foods.'

Evidence against my thought/Facts that discredit my thought:

'My thought doesn't have any scientific backing or evidence and is steeped in diet culture. There is no evidence to show that following this approach is good for my emotional and physical wellbeing. I haven't developed food neutrality yet and still demonize food which affects my approach to food.'

4. Reframe the thought: write down a compassionate and neutral thought.

'I understand that the more I restrict something, the more I want it, therefore I end up bingeing. It's important for me to develop food neutrality and I need to give myself unconditional permission to eat and stop depriving myself.'

5. Reflection.

'My 'should' statement is putting a lot of pressure on me and has its roots in diet culture. I'm going to spend more time working on food neutrality and developing unconditional permission with food.'

IDENTIFYING YOUR INNER FOOD CRITIC

Now that you've brought some awareness to how your inner food critic operates, we can start to characterize that voice a little more clearly. Take a moment to reflect on your inner food critic. What do they sound like? Are they an all-or-nothing thinker? Do they make you feel guilty for eating particular foods? Or try and convince you that you have to 'earn' foods? Do they catastrophize when you eat past comfortable fullness? You can recognize the inner food critic because they use words like 'should' and 'must'. Their tone is mean, cruel, and judgemental.

What about the advice they're giving you? Is your inner food critic saying things that are grounded in fads as opposed to something widely accepted and supported by scientific consensus? Did it come from a social media guru, or can you fact-check it from a reliable source? While there are always new studies and flashy headlines, promises of new superfoods and miracle diets, and anecdote upon anecdote of people online who claim to have cured themselves of all sorts of chronic conditions, credible nutrition advice hasn't changed that much, and isn't likely to do so.

On the flip side, think about what a more compassionate, caring voice – your *inner nurturer* – might sound like. How can you identify that voice? What words and phrases might they say to you? If you find it difficult to imagine this voice coming from within you, can you imagine the voice of a caring parent or other relative, a sibling, friend, or therapist? (Side note: I know some people don't like the term 'inner nurturer' – you could call them a coach or cheerleader instead. One of my clients would refer to her inner Wonder Woman – go with whatever feels good to you.)

Write down what your inner nurturer and inner critic sound like. What kind of things do they tell you?

Inner critic: **Inner nurturer:**

....

....

....

If you're finding it difficult to imagine what the voice of the inner critic and inner nurturer sound like, can you identify what they *look* like? Sometimes it's easier to visualize them – a bit like the devil and angel on your shoulder trope. For instance, a client of mine once drew a picture of her inner critic to look like a matted, tangled ball of deep purple yarn, while her inner nurturer was a beautiful garden full of spring flowers – a perfect metaphor for how the inner nurturer helps you grow and bloom.

In your journal, draw your inner critic and inner nurturer. Add as much detail as you can – colour, texture, shading, relative size, and so on

Your control centre

Imagine your mind has a control centre, with a host of different parts of you who all have a role to play in helping you navigate through life (anyone who has seen the film *Inside Out* knows what I'm talking about). Can you begin to notice when it's the inner critic calling the shots versus the inner nurturer? As you move through your day, notice when the inner critic is being particularly harsh or loud. Can you tune into what the inner nurturer might say instead? If it's helpful, write down a few key phrases or sentences that the inner nurturer might say that help you feel comforted when you're being judgemental about your body or critical of food choices or behaviours.

EXPANDING YOUR TOOLKIT

If you didn't feel like your toolkit was full enough, here are a few more you might want to add in! As with any of the tools, though, they're optional; it's important to find what's going to work for you!

Challenge accepted

This is a little challenge that we can use to try and shut down the inner food critic. So, whenever a sneaky diet mentality thought or food rule pops into your head, write it down. Then alongside it write **CHALLENGE ACCEPTED**, and go ahead and break the rule.

Afterwards, reflect on how the experience was:

* How did you feel?

* What happened?

* Were you able to eat and enjoy the food?

* Were there any consequences of eating the food, or is the world still standing?

Automatic negative thoughts

Sometimes the feelings of guilt and critical messages about certain foods are coming from within. These thoughts that pop up immediately after eating a cookie or whatever are known as automatic negative thoughts (ANTs). They're totally normal and a result of years of diet culture messages, but can be a total pain in the ass, especially when you want to chow down on a cookie in peace.

If we can mindfully identify thoughts as an ANT, then we can put a little distance between ourselves and the thoughts and look at them a little more objectively. We do this through 'the power of three' – three sentences or counterpoints to balance out the ANTs and help reframe them.

For example: The 'this cookie will make me fat' ANT becomes:

1 Maybe this cookie will satisfy my cravings, so I can stop thinking about food.

2 Eating a few cookies won't harm my health.

3 If I eat the cookie, I might realize it's not that big a deal.

Your turn: pick an ANT that you've had playing on repeat in your head:

Now write out your power of three, your three counterbalance points:

1 ....

2 ....

3 ....

Use your power of three next time you notice the inner critic being especially loud!

The false promise of the 'healthy alternative'

Diet and wellness culture teaches us that we should only be picking the most nutritionally optimal food possible – instead of having a regular slice of New York cheesecake, you feel pressure to make one out of raw nuts, dates, and coconut oil. Or say you fancy some cookie dough, and you find some wellness guru pushing their 'sugar free' version made with mashed chickpeas and carob nibs. I get that some people really like these types of recipes and are totally cool with them. But I'm willing to bet that for most of us they feel totally unsatisfying. Raise your hand if you've ever smashed twenty chocolate-covered rice cakes when you just want one Penguin? Exactly!

There's nothing inherently wrong with 'healthier' versions of foods. What I'm opposed to is that people often feel morally obligated to eat 'healthier' versions of foods that 1) aren't all that different in terms of nutritional value anyway, 2) don't taste as good as the real deal, 3) reinforce a food hierarchy, and 4) promote over-consumption of the 'healthier' version.

Have you ever told yourself any of the following?

* I can eat more because it's lower calorie.

* I'm allowed because it's 'clean'/all natural/unprocessed.

* It's healthier because it's refined-sugar free!

* It's a 'free food' so it doesn't count (then eaten fifty of said item).

 Can you think of a time you've applied this kind of logic to eating? Add some of your own examples – either recent or from the past – to the table opposite. This isn't about beating yourself up or judging yourself, but to help raise awareness of how the 'healthy' alternative may be colluding with your inner critic.

Craving	What I wanted to eat	What I actually ate	How I felt afterwards
Salty and sweet	Chocolate-covered pretzels	Whole family bag of salty and sweet 'skinny' popcorn	Stomach felt uncomfortable and weirdly full but empty at the same time – unsatisfied, short-changed
Comfort food	Mac and cheese with melted cheese on top	Cauliflower cheese then a little while later half a packet of biscuits	Should have just had pasta with some cauliflower on the side! Would probably still have wanted biscuits, but just enough to finish off meal

In the next chapter we'll work on leaning in to the pleasure and satisfaction of food but, for now, notice how the inner food critic undermines the intuitive eating process with the false economy of the 'healthy alternative.'

+ Do you find yourself overdoing it on healthy alternatives?
+ Do you feel pressure to always pick the 'healthiest' version of a food?
+ Has the healthy alternative kept you feeling restricted or deprived at all?

NAVIGATING NUTRITION INFORMATION

For every diet that exists, there are hundreds, if not thousands, of gurus, coaches, influencers, and journalists who want to give you their advice as to what constitutes a healthy food, diet, or relationship with food. A lot of these folks may be very well intentioned and just want to share a way of eating and living that works for them, but this doesn't always translate well into general advice. This phenomenon, of sharing your own experience as if it's a universal truth, is known as the 'n=1 effect'. In scientific studies the 'n' is the number of participants in a sample. Generally speaking, the greater the number of people you have in a study, the more 'power' the study has and the more likely we are to be able to identify links and patterns. In nutritional sciences in particular, the 'n' value of studies is usually in the 100s or 1000s – these studies are then repeated, often in different countries with different populations, to help us get a better idea of what is going on. This is the sort of information that we base our nutrition guidelines on: studies of the effects of diet in hundreds and thousands of people, not the opinion or experiences of one individual (or n=1). That's not to say that our experiences aren't all completely valid and important; they are. But when digesting this information, it's vital to recognize that what may work for your favourite Instagrammer won't necessarily work for you. This can be tricky to navigate when there is a seemingly endless barrage of highly clickable media articles and headlines about nutrition. It gives the impression that nutritional science is constantly evolving and changing and that scientists don't agree on anything. While there is plenty that's still up for debate, these are largely academic debates over minutiae rather than seismic shifts in the advice we have around nutrition. Periodically a client will send me a link to one of these media articles asking for my opinion on it. I will only very rarely click on the article, but I'll respond with some questions for the client to assess whether the article is helpful or harmful:

HOW TO JUST EAT IT

What was your intention behind clicking on the article? Was it motivated by self-care and self-compassion, or do you think it was rooted in fear and control? Do you think this article might reinforce the voice of the inner food critic? How do you think reading it might be helpful or harmful? Do you think it might trigger the diet mentality?

Next time you find yourself clicking on a flashy nutrition headline, reflect on the experience in your journal using these questions

My friends at The Rooted Project, registered dietitians Helen West and Rosie Saunt, put together this checklist to help you assess the quality of an article.

Red flags

☐ The headline makes bold or scary claims about food or a diet.

☐ It sounds too good to be true.

☐ It is written by a journalist, or 'health guru', who doesn't have specific training in nutrition. There's no expert quotes or input.

☐ It deals in absolutes or single approaches – eating a certain diet is the only way to achieve health, or the inclusion of certain foods will make you sick/healthy.

☐ It positions a single diet or a food as 'bad' or as a quick fix/cure-all.

Good signs

☐ The headline doesn't make claims about the health effects of a food or diet and isn't fear-promoting.

☐ The article is well balanced with a nuanced discussion of the topic, including uncertainties and unknowns.

☐ It was written by somebody with experience and training in the area being discussed (e.g. a registered nutritionist or dietitian or a nutritional scientist), or consults and quotes trained professionals.

☐ It recognizes that there's not one 'right' way to eat for everyone, and single foods, nutrients, or

Red flags

☐ It promotes the idea that our environment is toxic and that we need to only eat 'natural' foods or eat a certain way to cleanse or purify ourselves.

☐ The article is trying to sell you something, like a diet guide, supplement pill, or workout programme.

☐ The article focuses on body size as the measure of success for a way of eating.

Good signs

lifestyles aren't focused on as a way to gain or lose health.

☐ It recognizes diet as part of a much broader picture of health, which is influenced by complex physiological, psychological, social, and environmental factors.

☐ It doesn't promote ideas around single diets or foods being purifying or toxic.

☐ The article is not an advert, sponsored by a company selling products, or written by a person with a product to sell you.

☐ The article does not focus on weight change as the marker for achieving health.

Have you found yourself getting sucked into clickbait nutrition articles that promise to have all the answers?

How do they make you feel?

How do they collude with or reinforce the inner food critic?

Was clicking on the article motivated by self-care and compassion or fear and control?

Navigating media articles when you have a health concern

I appreciate that many of you who are reading this might be trying to manage a health concern like irritable bowel syndrome, polycystic ovary syndrome, or insulin resistance. This adds a layer of complexity to navigating media articles, as so often our concerns are trivialized or dismissed by healthcare professionals who are stumped for ways to help us, or aren't well-versed in Health at Every Size and intuitive eating paradigms and so may give us generic advice around 'losing weight' or 'eating healthily'. This can be enormously frustrating if you've tried every diet under the sun (and now you've read this book and know that's bad advice!), or you worry that restricting your diet could lead you back down the path of disordered eating and a difficult relationship with food. The good news is there are lots of wonderful dietitians and nutritionists who are sharing lots of advice and resources for managing your condition through a weight-inclusive and intuitive eating lens. Check out the resources at the back of the book. And at my clinic – London Centre for Intuitive Eating – we have provided a series of sliding scale guides to these conditions that are weight-inclusive and intuitive eating-aligned. They're designed for you to take to your doctor or other healthcare provider to help you advocate for the type of care you want. Go to gumroad.com/lcie to see the range of topics available.

+ Can I bring some mindful awareness to when the inner food critic is acting up?

+ What can I do or say to help me feel more grounded and not believe the stories the inner food critic is telling me?

+ Have I noticed any new fairy lights getting switched on?

+ Are there any tools from this section that you can add to your toolkit? Go back to Chapter 1 and write them in.

Listen to the corresponding podcast episode Don't Salt My Game – How to Just Eat It: Chapter 8

CHAPTER 8

MINDFUL EATING AND FINDING PLEASURE IN FOOD

For those with an eating disorder, mindful eating can sometimes increase or intensify ED thoughts and/or behaviours. Discuss mindful eating with your treatment team before tackling this section (although mindfulness in general might be a helpful tool to have in your recovery toolkit). Connection with the pleasure, joy and meaning in food can be a powerful tool for recovery if you feel ready.

OK, this is the part of intuitive eating where things start to get really exciting, where we can start to see food not as a source of conflict, but as a source of pleasure, joy, satisfaction, and creativity. Unlike the diet culture version of mindful eating, mindful eating in the context of intuitive eating is about *connecting with* and *exploring food*. It's about bringing *curiosity* to the experience of eating food, without *judgement*. It's about *noticing* how food feels in your mouth, mind, and body.

WHAT IS MINDFUL EATING?

Although not *technically* a principle of intuitive eating, I think the concept of mindful eating is super helpful when healing our relationship with food. However, if we come to mindful eating without having established a mindfulness practice, it can get dicey – we can end up using mindful eating as a way of trying to control our eating, which is not what it's about. Mindful eating is about getting curious about our experiences with food – whether they're positive, negative, or just neutral. The nitty-gritty of mindfulness is beyond the scope of this book, but there are loads of cool (and free) resources online. I really like mindful.org's getting started guide: mindful.org/meditation/mindfulness-getting-started/. Or you might prefer to try an app like *Headspace* or *Calm*. Once you've got into a good rhythm with mindfulness and feel like you've got the basics down (i.e. being with your experiences without judging them), then come back to this section on mindful eating practices.

Raisin meditation adapted from Jon Kabat-Zinn[1]

Elements of mindful eating

Jon Kabat-Zinn, the founder of Mindfulness Based Stress Reduction (MBSR), *the* guy in mindfulness, describes mindfulness as: 'The awareness that arises through paying attention, on purpose, non-judgementally, in the service of understanding and wisdom.' He's also the creator of the 'raisin meditation' – a mindful eating practice that gets you to tune into all of the sensory information being communicated when you eat something. In this instance, he picked a raisin, but if shrivelled old grapes aren't your deal, then you could pick just about any other small piece of food – a cashew nut or almond, a Smartie or Skittle, a raspberry, a piece of cheese. I think it's pretty interesting to do this activity with a raisin and then again with a grape to compare and contrast the two experiences.

Pick out the food you're going to use and if it's helpful, you can make notes to reflect on your experience

You can repeat this activity in your journal using different foods with different sensory qualities

Action	Notes/observations	Notes/observations
Holding	First, take a raisin and hold it in the palm of your hand or between your finger and thumb. Focusing on it, imagine that you've just dropped in from Mars and have never seen an object like this before in your life.	
Seeing	Take time to really see it; gaze at the raisin with care and full attention. Let your eyes explore every part of it, examining the highlights where the light shines, the darker hollows, the folds and ridges, and any asymmetries or unique features.	
Touching	Turn the raisin over between your fingers, exploring its texture, maybe with your eyes closed if that enhances your sense of touch.	
Smelling	Hold the raisin beneath your nose; with each inhalation drink in any smell, aroma, or fragrance that may arise, noticing as you do this anything interesting that may be happening in your mouth or stomach.	
Placing	Now slowly bring the raisin up to your lips, noticing how your hand and arm know exactly how and where to position it. Gently place the object in the mouth, without chewing, noticing how it gets into the mouth in the first place. Spend a few moments exploring the sensations of having it in your mouth, exploring it with your tongue.	
Tasting	When you are ready, prepare to chew the raisin, noticing how and where it needs to be for chewing. Then, very consciously, take one or two bites into it and notice what happens in the aftermath, experiencing any waves of taste that emanate from it as you continue chewing. Without swallowing yet, notice the sensations of taste and texture in the mouth and how these may change over time, moment by moment, as well as any changes in the object itself.	

HOW TO JUST EAT IT

Action	Notes/observations	Notes/observations
Swallowing	When you feel ready to swallow the raisin, see if you can first detect the intention to swallow as it comes up, so that even this is experienced consciously before you actually swallow the raisin.	
Following	Finally, see if you can feel what is left of the raisin moving down into your stomach, and sense how the body as a whole is feeling after completing this exercise in mindful eating.	

Mindful eating meditation

Similarly to the hunger body scan in Chapter 3, I want you to record this mindful eating practice on your phone and play it back to yourself (or ask a friend to do it for you). I've written this to be used with chocolate: an individual Quality Street or Celebration would be perfect. But if you're not a chocolate person, you can write out your own script using the following as a template but mixing it up to describe the food you're going to eat. Pizza, yoghurt-covered almonds, ice cream, crisps, cherries, whatever.

Get yourself nice and comfortable . . . Take a few deep breaths, in through your nose and out through your mouth . . .

Now look at the chocolate in your hand, notice the shiny foil . . . Are there any patterns or designs on the wrapper?

Gently closing your eyes, move the chocolate around in your hands . . . Rub your fingers over the foil and feel the textures and shape of the chocolate underneath . . . can you trace any ridges or designs on the chocolate itself? Feel the weight of the chocolate, is it dense or is it light? Imagine what's inside the foil . . . smooth, rich chocolate that will melt when you put it in your mouth . . . Maybe there's caramel in the middle or maybe it has notes of orange or vanilla . . . perhaps there are some nuts or crunchy pieces inside . . .

Record the script on your phone and play it back to yourself

For now just imagine what it's going to taste like as you bite into it . . . Is it hard, or soft and melty? Is it solid or filled in the centre?

Now, open your eyes and gently peel back the foil . . . listen to the sound of the foil crinkling as you unwrap it . . . Take a look at the chocolate underneath . . . Gaze at it as though you've never seen a chocolate like this before.

What do you see? How would you describe the chocolate? Is it textured or patterned, or completely smooth? What colour is it? . . . Is it rich and dark, or milky and creamy? . . .

Anticipate the flavours in your mouth . . . Are they smooth, or are they sharp and bitter?

Now lift the chocolate up to your nose and take a deep breath in . . . What do you smell? Notice all the different scents that go into the chocolate . . . Does it smell sweet? . . . Can you pick out different scents? Vanilla, cocoa, maybe butterscotch or honey, brown sugar, orange blossom, or mint . . .

Notice any sensations that you might experience in your mouth, stomach, or elsewhere in your body.

Now it's time to take a bite of the chocolate, but don't chew it yet . . . Let the flavours melt into your tongue . . . What do you taste? . . . What flavours are present? . . . Is it the same as what you expected?

What are the textures you feel? . . . How does it feel on your tongue as you slowly roll it around your mouth? . . . Does the flavour change over time or as you slowly begin to chew? . . . Does it get stuck on your teeth or on the roof of your mouth?

When you're ready, go ahead and swallow. Notice the sensation on the back of your tongue travelling down towards your stomach . . . How does it feel in your stomach and elsewhere in your body?

HOW TO JUST EAT IT

Now take a second and third bite. Does the chocolate change flavours? Is it as good as the first bite?

It can be nice to repeat this activity every now and then with your favourite snack. I often tell clients to think of it as some self-care alone time and to find themselves some peace and quiet, even just for five or ten minutes to have a cup of tea and a bite to eat.

Bringing more mindfulness to the eating experience

Eating 100 per cent mindfully at every single meal might not be feasible or practical for us (and we don't need that kind of pressure in our lives). But is it possible to bring elements of mindful eating to the eating experience – even in small or subtle ways? Here are some ideas for you to consider; circle the ones that feel doable for you or that you'd like to try out.

* Putting my phone on Do Not Disturb.

* Closing my laptop or moving away from my desk to have my meal/snack.

* Committing to one mindful bite at the beginning and end of my meal/snack.

* Setting aside 15 minutes to put my feet up and mindfully enjoy a snack.

* Noticing the shapes, colours, textures, aromas, and consistencies of ingredients transform as I cook.

* Picking one mindful eating element from this chapter to focus on when eating (i.e. texture, temperature, or seeing/following).

* Bringing a sense of gratitude for the Deliveroo guy.

THE PLEASURE PRINCIPLE

A lot of us might feel a bit threatened by the idea of food being pleasurable – it might have become conflated with diet culture's idea of 'indulgent', 'decadent', and of course the classic 'guilty pleasure'. All of these are code words for 'being bad' and 'breaking your diet'. These types of foods are only permissible at Christmas, Easter, and birthdays. The rest of the time, if we choose to eat these foods then we have to pay penance in the form of more exercise, restriction, feelings of shame, or most often all three. When we restrict and deprive ourselves of these foods, though, the pendulum is more likely to swing into doughnutland, right? So discovering which foods give us most pleasure, and therefore most satisfaction, can help us tune into what we really want to eat and what will leave us feeling content and comfortably full. Remember the activity on The False Promise of the 'Healthy Alternative' (page 215) – when we are following rules-based eating, or dieting, we might feel pressure to get as much 'bang for our buck' as possible to try and appease feelings of deprivation. We've all been there – a whole carton of low-calorie ice cream instead of a few scoops of Cookie Dough ice cream. Twenty rice cakes instead of one packet of crisps. A cauliflower 'pizza' instead of the real deal. Chances are we eat way more of these so-called healthy alternatives than what we really want or need in order to satisfy our cravings. But these foods tend to be missing the essential ingredients that make food enjoyable – fat, salt, sugar, carbs! So we never feel content eating them and never get to satisfy our cravings.

We may also force ourselves to eat foods that we think are 'healthy' or 'good for us' – baby carrots and low-fat hummus, anyone? – but that aren't all that satisfying, propagating the cycle of deprivation. Look, hummus needs fat. And probably also some toasted pitta bread or crunchy breadsticks to elevate it from diet snack to super satisfying snack. The difference between the two is how much pleasure we derive from eating it. So we're going to spend some time really digging into what gives us the most pleasure, satisfaction, and contentment from the foods we eat from a sensory perspective. Because intuitive eating is all about eating with our senses as opposed to eating according to rules.

To start with, grab your food icons (appendix, page 313) and lay them all out in front of you. It's best if you can do this when you're a little bit hungry. Close your eyes for a moment and consider the different foods – to which ones does your mind immediately gravitate, which ones make your mouth water, which make your belly grumble a little, which ones do you feel excited about eating? Pull out the foods that you'd really like to eat – try and pick as many as you can so you have a big sample to work with.

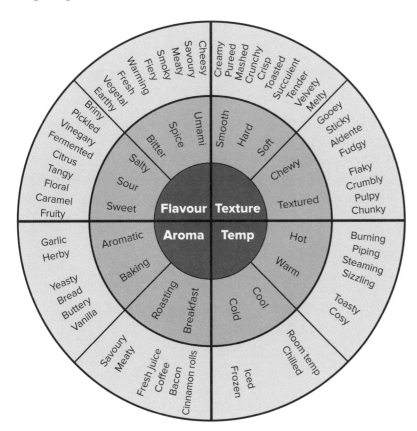

Now, using the sensory wheel to help, do you notice any patterns in the foods you picked out in terms of textures, flavours, aromas or temperatures that come up? Can you group any of these foods together in interesting ways that don't reinforce a good/bad dichotomy? For instance, 'crispy' may include a fresh green apple, ready salted crisps, bacon, ginger snaps, and iceberg lettuce leaves. Keep playing around and find different ways of categorizing the foods according to different sensory components.

Now, using the sensory wheel and your food icons, answer the following questions to help discover which elements bring you the most joy, pleasure, and satisfaction

Flavour

✷ Which flavours do you gravitate most towards?

✷ Does that change throughout the day? For instance, are you more of a sweet or savoury breakfast person?

✷ Do you like to mix flavours or do you prefer to keep it pretty simple?

✷ What do your flavour preferences tell you about the type(s) of cuisine you like to eat?

✷ Do you like big and bold or more subtle and nuanced flavours?

✷ Do you like combos or contrasts of flavour, like sweet and salty? Or do you like one unifying flavour?

✷ Are there any flavours you really don't like?

✷ Do these flavours remind you of a specific time, place, or person? Like a holiday or a time of year?

Texture

* Which textures do you gravitate most towards?

* Are there any you dislike?

* Does your texture preference change throughout the day?

* Do you get bored eating 'samey' textures in one meal?

* Can you experiment with having different textures in your meals?

* Do you associate any of these textures with a memorable meal you've eaten or another special memory?

Temperature

* Which foods do you enjoy eating when they're cool or very cold (hello frozen cheesecake!)?

* Which foods do you prefer to eat warmed up? (Like a toasted teacake, for instance.)

* How about foods that you prefer to be sizzling hot?

* Piping-hot stews, steaming mugs of tea, and bowls of soup are great in the winter; but what about when the weather is warmer? Do you like ice cream, watermelon, and crisp salads?

* Do you like cold food straight out of the fridge or hot food that's sizzling? Or does it taste better once it has come to room temperature?

* Do you prefer hot or cold breakfasts? What about lunch and dinner?

Aroma

* Are there any scents or aromas that especially stand out to you?

* Are there any scents that you strongly dislike?

* What information can this give you about the types of foods you like to eat and which foods will provide lots of pleasure?

* Do these aromas remind you of a specific time, place, or person? Like a holiday or a time of year?

The following elements aren't in the sensory wheel but are just as important to consider when it comes to pleasure and satisfaction.

Variety

Not every meal can be mezze or tapas-style, but think about how you can change things up throughout the week. Also think about how you can add a little interesting variety to your everyday meals with some different sauces, toppings, and garnishes. Variety can help us make sure we're covering all our bases nutritionally, but having options also means your taste buds won't get bored!

* Do you tend to eat the same thing day in, day out?

* Or do you like to mix it up and get creative?

* How could you add more variety to meals?

Appearance

OK, so it doesn't have to be Insta-worthy, but putting a little effort into presentation can help with the satisfaction factor. Think about colourful garnishes, pretty bowls for different sauces or condiments on the side, breaking up 'samey' foods with a little something to jazz it up. Think about how you can make meals a bit more interesting to look at. Here are some ideas:

* Do you have a variety of textures and flavours? Imagine a plate of chicken, mashed potatoes, and cauliflower; it's all the same boring beige food. You could make it fresher by swapping the cauliflower for some crisp salad. You could roast the potatoes or make wedges with some tasty seasoning.

* Garnishes are really quick and easy and can make a big impact: herbs like chives or coriander, sesame seeds, spices like sumac or chilli flakes, a good-quality table salt like Maldon, cracked black pepper, sauerkraut, or pickled veg.

* Sauces/dips: ketchup, tahini dressing, soy sauce, guacamole, fruit chutney, hummus, wholegrain mustard, hot sauce, tzatziki.

Experience

Are you eating standing up, straight out of the fridge? Or do you take time to set the table and sit down and eat mindfully? Are you eating at your computer? With the TV on? Or while aimlessly scrolling through your phone? How many of your meals are eaten while you are distracted? How can you make sure you're not distracted while eating (with the goal of increasing the satisfaction or pleasure of a meal and knowing when you're full and ready to stop eating).

DON'T GET IT TWISTED

Tapping into pleasure, satisfaction, contentment, and the joy of food doesn't mean that every meal or snack will be *perfect* and totally hit the spot. That's too much pressure. Sometimes we have to smash a granola bar in our faces between meetings to keep us going; remember that honouring your hunger is the foundation of intuitive eating. To me at least, it's far more important to eat when you're feeling hunger pangs than to try and stave off hunger in order to find the 'perfect' thing to eat. The reality is that some eating experiences will be disappointing – sometimes you have to eat your mother-in-law's crappy stew, sometimes you have to eat a cold dinner after the kids have gone to bed, sometimes you only have enough money to buy a lacklustre supermarket sandwich until you get paid. None of this is 'wrong', it's not 'failing' at intuitive eating. What's worth remembering, though, is that unlike with dieting and rules-based eating, you are not condemned to these sub-par foods at every eating occasion. If a meal or snack is pretty *meh*, that's OK, because you know you can swing by the shop on the way home and get something tasty. Or if you're sick of eating the same leftovers from the past couple of days, you can take comfort in an interesting or exciting dessert.

> Notice if you are trying to perfect your meals. This is common after long periods of dieting and restriction – now you're a lot closer to food freedom, why wouldn't you want to maximize every food experience? What would help you sit with those less than perfect eating experiences?

CONNECTING WITH FOOD

I once had a client tell me that she hadn't been in a supermarket in over two years. She did all her shopping online, and bought the same foods every week (she was on a strict diet). While ordering online is super convenient, especially if it's physically difficult for you to get to the shops, it really narrows down our experience of food. When we are caught up in diet culture, our experience with food is reduced to two things: eating, or trying to stop ourselves from eating. The world of food has so much more to offer than that. Food is culture, tradition, history, creativity, entertainment, love and relationships.

Look, nobody is telling you to become a *foodie* (although go for it, if that's your jam), but thinking about connecting with food in other ways can be a powerful approach to healing your relationship with food.

Think about how you currently connect or engage with food – are you thinking about food purely as fuel, or as something to be conquered, or is food more of a creative endeavour or hobby? Here are some ways that clients have started exploring and connecting with food – do any resonate for you? Add more of your own, if you can.

* Spending a Saturday afternoon at the market, picking up the produce and feeling if it's ripe, tasting the cheese samples, smelling the fresh bread.

* Learning about different cultures' cuisines (from people who belong to that culture) – online or from a book.

* Growing a garden or even just growing some herbs on your windowsill.

* Kitchen experiments – fermenting, bread baking, pickling.

* Watching food documentaries/shows – some favourites include: *Salt, Fat, Acid, Heat, Chef's Table, Ugly Delicious*.

* Exploring a new restaurant in your town that you wouldn't normally go to.

* Baking a cake from a packet and licking the bowl afterwards.

* Asking your nan to teach you her favourite recipe (bonus if it's a family secret).

* Carpet picnics with the kids.

* Cooking for or with someone you care about.

* Learning how to prepare something simple from scratch.

* Giving yourself permission to play with food and get your hands dirty.

* Teaching kids about food (there are some great food encyclopedias with pictures of foods from all over the world), or playing shop with empty food cartons.

* ....

* ....

* ....

+ In what ways do you currently connect with food?

+ Do you avoid food outside of either eating or trying to stop yourself from eating? Is there anything you could do from the list above to connect more with food?

+ Does learning about food help enhance your enjoyment?

SUPERMARKET VISUALIZATION

This is a little thought experiment to help you visualize what you might buy at a supermarket that had anything and everything you could ever want to eat, and if money was no object. This is total fantasy and unrealistic for most of us, especially anyone on a strict food budget or living with food insecurity. The intention here is not that we will go out and buy all this stuff, but that we notice areas where we might be depriving ourselves, or where we can tap into what might bring us pleasure and satisfaction, particularly if we have been stuck deciding what to eat.

Adapted from
Susie Orbach

Record the following script on your phone and then play it back. As you imagine yourself moving through the imaginary supermarket, you can make a note of what you'd put in your shopping basket using the sections below. Make sure to include the pauses (. . .) in order to give yourself enough time to reflect and write down what you're picking out from the relevant supermarket section.

Imagine yourself standing in your kitchen . . . You open up the cupboards and the fridge; there isn't much there apart from a packet of rice cakes, and some kale that's starting to go off. Your kitchen is bare. How does this make you feel?. . . Are you comforted by the thought of having no food around you, or does it trigger a deprivation mindset? . . .

You decide you need to do a shop and fill up the kitchen with delicious and satisfying foods; you have an unlimited budget and you need to make sure the kitchen is really well stocked. You go to the food hall in your favourite high-end department store; it has everything you could ever want to eat under one roof . . . There's a bakery where everything is made fresh each day, a butcher with high-quality meat and fish, a deli counter with delicious prepared foods, a cheesemonger, an icecream counter, a smoothie bar, a pizza oven, fresh sushi, a

Make sure you're sitting somewhere comfortable where you won't be disturbed, with your journal and a pen to make notes

MINDFUL EATING AND FINDING PLEASURE IN FOOD

Write down your shopping list from each imaginary supermarket section; we'll use this in the reflections activity below

greengrocer, a make-your-own burrito stand, a salad and hot food bar, and everything in between . . .

You don't need to know the exact meals you're going to make or quantities or anything like that – this is just a low-stress way for you to imagine all the food that you might like to try. You grab a trolley, and start working your way around the shop, stopping to pick items up and examine them before putting them in your trolley.

You start in the bakery section. There are fresh sourdough breads, still hot from the oven, flaky croissants, and Portuguese custard tarts that are gently browned on top . . . There are eclairs with fresh cream, and a whole chocolate fudge cake . . . There's rosemary and olive oil focaccia with sea salt, and bagels with every seasoning . . . There are cinnamon buns drizzled in icing and everything else you'd expect from a quality bakery . . . Stop and note down in your journal what you pick up in the bakery section . . .

Now move on to the meat counter (if you're veggie, skip this part): tender steaks, wild-caught Scottish smoked salmon, pork and apple sausages. Make a note of what sounds good in this section . . .

Next it's the deli counter: smoked hummus, caramelized onion hummus, beetroot hummus, any kind of hummus you can imagine, golden falafel and pickled turnip that has turned bright pink, garlic-stuffed olives, chorizo, sun-blushed tomatoes, artichokes, honey-roasted ham, salami, prosciutto . . . List what you're going to pick up at the deli . . .

On to the cheesemonger: Brie, Parmesan, Camembert, Gruyère, Morbier, tangy mature Cheddar, halloumi, Jarlsberg, Stilton and any other type of cheese you can imagine. Pause and reflect on what you pick up from the cheese counter and add it to your list . . .

Next up is the greengrocer: bright red cherries on the stem, soft juicy peaches that smell like heaven, soft ripe avocados, vine-ripened

HOW TO JUST EAT IT

tomatoes, Tenderstem broccoli, bright pink radishes and ruby-red strawberries, golden-yellow corn still on the cob, emerald-green baby spinach leaves, sunny sweet potatoes and humble white ones . . . List the items you pick up in the greengrocer section . . .

Continue through the whole shop like this, section by section, adding foods to your trolley . . . Dry goods, frozen foods, the salad and hot food bar, the sushi counter, the smoothie and juice bar, the pizza oven, where you can pick your own toppings and take home a hot, fresh pizza, the taco and burrito station, and the ice cream and gelato bar, plus anything else you can imagine; make sure you write everything down . . .

{long pause to allow yourself time to write everything down}

Now imagine making your way home and stocking your cupboards, fridge, biscuit tin, fruit bowl, freezer, everything. Take a look around at your kitchen now. How does it feel to have an abundance of foods? Do you feel content knowing that there are plenty of delicious foods available? Or does it feel overwhelming? What would you need to feel safe? Can you relax, safe in the knowledge that food will always be available to you? If it still feels a little scary, can you think of anything that is comforting or soothing about being around the food? Do you feel the scarcity mindset loosening its grip?

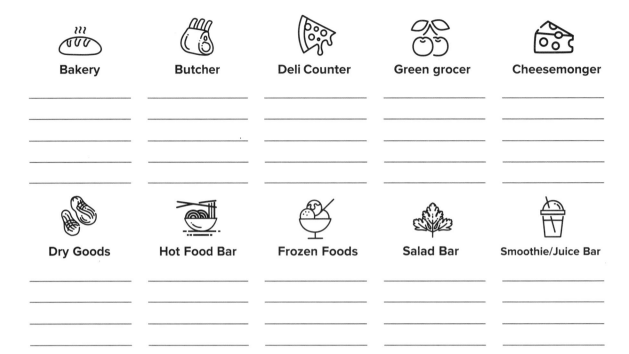

Bakery

_____
_____
_____
_____
_____

Butcher

_____
_____
_____
_____
_____

Deli Counter

_____
_____
_____
_____
_____

Green grocer

_____
_____
_____
_____
_____

Cheesemonger

_____
_____
_____
_____
_____

Dry Goods

_____
_____
_____
_____
_____

Hot Food Bar

_____
_____
_____
_____
_____

Frozen Foods

_____
_____
_____
_____
_____

Salad Bar

_____
_____
_____
_____
_____

Smoothie/Juice Bar

_____
_____
_____
_____
_____

✚ Did you notice anything interesting or surprising doing this activity?

✚ What does it tell you about areas where you might not be allowing yourself unconditional permission?

✚ Does your usual shopping contain a lot of the things you picked out in this imaginary supermarket?

✚ Or are there any foods that you typically buy but didn't pick up here – and does that tell you anything about what you think you 'should' be eating?

✚ Did you get a lot of balance in this shopping trolley overall – not just in terms of the types of foods, but also the flavours and textures and variety?

TASTE TEST

Sometimes feeling physically nourished is about rounding your meal out with something tasty. This could literally be anything: a spoonful of Nutella, some cheese and biscuits, a bunch of grapes, a cup of tea and some biscuits, a yoghurt, whatever. But people invariably say that to round out a meal, they just want a square or two of dark chocolate or something else that is diet-y/wellness. And before you start proclaiming how much you love dark chocolate, just let this percolate for a second. Do you love dark chocolate because you love its bitter complexity on your tongue? Or do you love it because diet culture has taught you it's healthier, better for you, and has antioxidants or something?

Fine, some people genuinely love dark chocolate, and that's cool. But let's dig a little deeper with this one – do you really love dark chocolate that much? Or has diet culture convinced you that it's somehow superior? Do you get your kicks from rice cakes and skinny popcorn? Or do they leave you feeling short-changed and less than satisfied? There's nothing wrong with these foods – no judgement, remember? Whatever floats your boat, we're cool with. But what we want to help you get to the bottom of is whether you legitimately enjoy these foods – or has diet culture convinced you that you should like them?

Doing a side-by-side comparison of some of these foods can be a great way to figure out if you really do enjoy them. Think about a food that you enjoy in both its diet/wellness form and the not-so-wellness form, for example dark vs milk chocolate, rice cakes vs regular crisps. Use the worksheet below to taste each food and write your thoughts under each of the different pleasure aspects to help you decide which one you prefer.

Test food 1:	Test food 2:
Flavour:	Flavour:
Texture:	Texture:
Aroma:	Aroma:
Appearance:	Appearance:
Experience:	Experience:
Rate satisfaction ___ / 10	Rate satisfaction ___ / 10

+ Have you discovered any areas where you were depriving yourself of pleasure and satisfaction around food?

+ Have any more fairy lights switched on for you?

+ How does it feel to reframe food as something for discovery and exploration, rather than something to micromanage?

+ Are there any tools from this section that you can add to your toolkit? Go back to Chapter 1 and write them in).

CHAPTER 9
FEELING YOUR FULLNESS

Listen to the corresponding podcast episode Don't Salt My Game – How to Just Eat It: Chapter 9

Feeling our fullness is an important concept in intuitive eating. When we've been in the diet mentality for a long time, we may be afraid of letting ourselves feel full, either because we associate it with 'blowing' our diet, or because we associate fullness with physical and emotional discomfort.

As I've said, people have a tendency to equate intuitive eating with 'the hunger and fullness diet'. They hone in on just these elements of intuitive eating, forgetting that there's a whole lot more that goes into this process. If you've found yourself flicking straight to this section to try and learn how you can stop yourself from eating 'too much', cool your jets. You *have* to do the work. These principles do not exist as discrete entities that you can check off one by one. So if you haven't spent time with the other concepts, please slow down and go back. You might even find that by working your way through those other concepts, fullness takes care of itself, without you having to overthink it. This is because when the threat of deprivation is high, our ability to tune into and respect our bodies is low (remember the dietland to doughnutland pendulum). So we have to fully and completely work our way out of deprivation and restriction before fullness will 'click' for us – remember, our bodies need to learn to trust we will provide them with satisfying foods on a regular basis.

For those with an eating disorder, the fullness gauge can sometimes be broken and unreliable, making you feel fuller before you're truly filled up. It's essential to follow your treatment team's advice about how much you need to be eating. But learning that fullness isn't a bad thing can also be helpful, so proceed with caution.

WHAT IS FULLNESS?

In the same way that 'overweight' and 'ob*se' are loaded with judgement and stigma, I've found the word 'overeating' to be troubling. It reinforces the idea that there's a perfect point at which we should stop eating, and anything over that is 'bad'. This is, of course, not true. The point of comfortable fullness varies from day to day and meal to meal. How much food it takes to help us feel full will depend on the last time we ate, the type of food we are eating, and how satisfying a food is. I highly recommend removing 'overeating' from your vocabulary. Instead try using terms like 'comfortable fullness' and 'eating past comfortable fullness'; they're a lot less judgemental.

WHAT IS A 'NORMAL' SERVING SIZE?

Diet culture teaches us to eat like little birds, and then teaches us to feel like shit if we eat more than that. I call this *reverse portion distortion*. We hear about how serving sizes in restaurants have increased over time (and I'm not denying this), but at the same time, our idea of what is an appropriately satisfying portion *for us* has become so warped and skewed by diet culture, we don't seem to recognize that we actually need to eat a considerable amount of food to feel satisfied. Or, if we do eat to satisfaction, we judge ourselves hard. So we turn to the portion size advice on food packaging for reassurance. The difficulty is, this is somewhat arbitrary, being dictated by the food industry to fit particular standards for making claims about their products. For people in recovery (whether from an eating disorder, disordered eating, or diet culture) portion sizes can get in the way of us nourishing our bodies in a way that is truly satisfying. We may end up taking smaller sizes than what we actually need to help us feel content, reinforcing the 'forbidden fruit' effect and fuelling food preoccupation. Portion sizes undermine the trust we have in our bodies by making us overthink everything we eat, with the effect of being stuck in our heads. It's yet another tool diet culture uses to keep us disconnected from our bodies.

So how do you know what a portion is for you? Well, there are no hard and fasts, but the following might give you some clues. A serving size is based on:

* How hungry you are

* When you last ate

* How satisfying you find a food

* When you will eat again

* How something tastes

* Your access to food

* How you feel emotionally

* How filling a food is

Have you found yourself turning food packaging portion sizes into a rule? Do you let them dictate how much you're 'allowed' to eat? How have external portion size references made you feel — especially when you have eaten more than what the label suggests?

OBJECTIVE VS SUBJECTIVE BINGEING

'Binge' is another word that gets thrown around without much care or attention. We all *think* we know what binge eating is, but the reality is often very different from the picture that diet culture paints, where 'binge eating' is half a tub of Ben and Jerry's after a Domino's on a Saturday night. This can subjectively feel like more food than is comfortable – although for a lot of folks, this is just a regular Saturday night and no biggie (see, for example, my husband).

Through the lens of diet culture, and in the context of restriction, however, eating past comfortable fullness on a regular basis might be a symptom of disordered eating. Use the following table to help define and put into perspective the differences between objective and subjective bingeing.

Objective		Subjective	
Distressing	✓	Distressing	
Accompanied by a mix of feelings, such as guilt, shame, comfort, numbing out, or dissociation		Accompanied by feelings of guilt and shame	
A symptom of an eating disorder		A symptom of disordered eating	
Eating more food than most people might eat in an entire day in a short period of time (like 2 hours)		Eating more food than diet culture deems appropriate	
Ritualized and planned in advance (going to the shop specifically to buy binge foods)		A by-product of restriction and deprivation – whether physical, mental, or emotional	
Very difficult to stop a binge if someone else walked into the room		May feel out of control, but it's likely that if someone were to walk into the room you'd be able to stop and walk away from the food	

Objective		Subjective	
Associated with enormous physical discomfort that may last several hours		Associated with mild physical discomfort that usually passes within around 30 minutes to one hour	
May or may not be accompanied by purging behaviours like vomiting, restriction, laxative or diuretic use, or intense physical activity		May be accompanied by compensatory behaviours like 'being good' and doing an extra workout the next day	
A coping mechanism		A coping mechanism	

✚ Have you noticed a connection between restriction/dieting and bingeing (either objective or subjective)?

✚ What impact has diet culture had on your perception of how much food is 'acceptable' to eat?

✚ Has diet culture distorted the idea of what a binge really is?

WHAT DOES COMFORTABLE FULLNESS FEEL LIKE?

Just like the hunger body scan in Chapter 3, you can use the following checklist to help you be curious about your own subjective sense of fullness. These correspond with the 'comfortably full' section of the hunger wheel on page 104, use your cut out and keep version in the appendix to explore these sensations.

Mood	Energy	Head	Stomach	Body
content	recharged	improved concentration	comfortable	no longer interested in food
calm	energized*	focused	gently full	food no longer makes you salivate
happy	sleepy	clear	slightly bloated/burpy	reduced cravings
satisfied			gurgling/ digesting	eating slows down
sated				

* When we eat we may notice a change in our energy levels. Initially we might feel a little bit sleepy after eating a meal as our body is digesting it, but we will likely overall feel more energized by eating. Food, after all, is what creates energy in our bodies

Can you circle the elements in this table that signal fullness before and after eating a snack?

THE FULLNESS GAP

Somewhere I see people get a bit stuck with intuitive eating is when they stop eating when they're no longer hungry, but not yet full. Think about that for a second. There's a period while eating where you're not super hungry any more, but the tank isn't all the way filled up either – maybe around a 5 or 6 on the hunger and satisfaction guide. Think of it like juicing your phone battery up to 50 or 60 per cent. Sure, it'll keep you going for a while, but sooner or later you're going to hit low power mode. Sometimes we only want a little top-up to keep us going until dinner (aka a snack), but more often I see people fall into the fullness gap because they're afraid of fullness. Ironically, it's not allowing ourselves to feel all the way full that keeps us thinking about and being preoccupied with food. Remember that fullness is not a pathology. We are not sheep; we have not evolved to spend eighteen hours a day chomping grass (I don't know how long sheep actually spend eating, don't @ me). The point is, allowing our bellies to fully fill up ensures we have enough physical and mental energy to keep us doing the things we find truly fulfilling.

The difference between fullness and satisfaction

Another potentially tricky concept to grasp is the difference between fullness and satisfaction. Fullness tends to be physical, whereas satisfaction is perhaps more psychological. Technically you can fill up on anything, right? You could drink a bottle of olive oil and feel full, but I'm guessing that's not such a satisfying eating experience. We need both fullness *and* satisfaction to feel 'done' with a meal or snack. Likewise, you might have a bite of *the* most delicious chocolate fudge brownie in the world, but if it's not enough to be filling then chances are you'll be left wanting more. The difference between fullness and satisfaction will vary from person to person, but here are some ideas:

* Eating balanced meals that contain a mixture of proteins, fats, and carbs (and don't scrimp on any of these components).

* Making sure there's always a 'fun food' element to your meals – something you're looking forward to and will enjoy – again this is subjective.

* Adding toppings or sauces to a meal that would otherwise be kinda boring – cheese, sour cream, guacamole, salsa, croutons, salad dressing.

* Or a tasty side – fresh bread and butter, tortilla chips with a bowl of chilli.

* Dessert! Apple crumble and custard, fruit and yoghurt with honey, Nutella or peanut butter straight from the jar, a bunch of cold red grapes, cookies, cake, a bowl of granola, cheese and biscuits. Don't be constrained by limited definitions of 'dessert' – it can be whatever helps you feel content and satisfied.

✚ What makes the difference between fullness and satisfaction for you? Write down some words you associate with each.

✚ Have you noticed yourself ever falling into the fullness gap?

✚ How do you know you're eating enough and not becoming a victim of reverse portion distortion?

✚ How can you practise kindness if you find that you've eaten past comfortable fullness?

✚ Are there any tools from this section that you can add to your toolkit? Go back to Chapter 1 and write them in.

Listen to the corresponding podcast episode Don't Salt My Game – How to Just Eat It: Chapter 10

CHAPTER 10

INTUITIVE MOVEMENT

For those with an eating disorder, movement can be another manifestation of the disorder, so it's important to unpack this as part of your recovery. If possible, it can be helpful to take a complete break from movement and come back to it when you have found some more balance and can approach it from a place of curiosity rather than as an obligation to the ED.

Intuitive movement is about finding joy in activity, whether it's taking a low-impact yoga class, going for a walk, or training for a marathon – finding an activity that doesn't leave you drained and exhausted is a critical part of the process. Working out what is enjoyable for you, rather than what a diet or healthy lifestyle plan dictates, will make it more sustainable in the long run than those intense exercise routines that you can't keep up with. This stage of IE is about helping you explore all the shades of grey in finding joyful, sustainable forms of movement. Let's start by taking a deeper look at what intuitive movement is and how we can use it to guide us to finding more pleasure in our bodies.

What is intuitive movement?

Tally Rye,
Personal trainer and
author of *Train Happy*
@tallyrye

Intuitive movement is the practice of building trust with your body so you can make the right decisions as to which type of movement is best for you – along with the right decisions about intensity, duration and rest.

In the same way as you have applied the principles of intuitive eating to your relationship with food, we need to do the same for our relationship with fitness.

For many of us who are recovering from diet culture, exercise has been closely linked to restriction, punishment, and earning and burning food. Diet culture co-opted the fitness industry and made us think its sole purpose was body and weight manipulation, and so it became a chore that we 'had' to endure. Many of us struggle to separate it from these damaging ideas. The good news is that exercise is not just a tool for body and weight manipulation; it can be so much more.

We have work to do to untangle the idea that exercise is just a tool of weight loss and aesthetics. We can use the process of intuitive movement to find joy in moving our bodies while feeling more at home and connected with ourselves. This can help us to have a sustainable and happy relationship with movement.

Let's look at the principles of intuitive eating and apply them to how we approach fitness.

Reject the diet mentality: This is about shifting the intention behind movement and finding your own intrinsic motivation to move. Start by acknowledging the negative impact that weight-centric fitness has had, and make a conscious decision to let movement become about joy, self-care, community, and a fun physical challenge. Curate your social media to reflect this; unfollow the diet culture #fitspos and follow diverse accounts that show joyful movement in a variety of ways and by a variety of people. I recommend @meg.boggs, @kanoagreene, @jonelleyoga, @missfitsworkout, @sophjbutler, and @fatgirlshiking.

Also consider ditching the diet culture tools: take a break from fitness watches, progress pictures, scales, and measurements.

Honour your exercise appetite and stop when satisfied: Work on building awareness of your body's appetite to move and of when you need to rest. These questions help:

✖ How would you like to move your body?

✖ How energetic do you feel today?

✖ When do you want to move? What time of day feels best?

✖ How long do you want to exercise for?

✖ When is your body asking for rest? What are those signals?

Listening to your body's answers to these questions will allow you to begin to engage in exercise on your *own* terms. Honouring your body's needs for rest and movement will strengthen the sense of trust, and signals will become increasingly clearer.

Make peace with exercise: Diet culture taught us that there are 'good' and 'bad' foods; well, it did the same with types of fitness. For example, many of us think super sweaty cardio workouts are 'good', because of the underlying narrative that 'good' exercise is about calorie burn, and low-intensity workouts like yoga are 'bad', because they don't exhaust the body in the same way.

But guess what? Neither is better than the other, as all forms of movement have their place. It's less about what the workout is, and more about the intention behind the workout. And as we shift to a place of movement for self-care, that will inform the exercise choices we make – not the calorie burn!

Challenge the fitness police: Through diet culture, many of us have created a set of rules about working out. Perhaps you feel that you have to work out for a certain amount of time and at a certain level of intensity? Or that you must complete a certain number of sessions a week, and never miss a Monday? Ask yourself where these rules came from, and how they make you feel about exercise – and challenge them. For example, you might tell yourself you 'must' work out for 60 minutes in the gym, when actually you feel satisfied with shorter workouts that last 20–30 minutes. So honour that, and do what feels best for you.

Discover the feel good factor: Exercise is no longer a form of punishment, and should not be motivated by guilt and shame. Instead, approach movement as a form of self-care, self-respect, and self-expression. Focus on how good your chosen activities make you feel: proud, strong, confident, powerful, connected to yourself, and part of a community.

Managing emotions: Movement can be a therapeutic tool to help us build inner strength and resilience. This helps us dig deeper into our feelings and emotions. It is important to state that it should not be used instead of therapy or medication, but as a supporting tool alongside those things. This can include slowing down on sad days and connecting with emotion through a yoga sequence, putting boxing gloves on and punching out the stress, or getting outside in nature to gain some perspective on life. We often use exercise as a means to avoid emotions, but an intuitive approach is about acknowledging and working with them.

Accepting your body: Contrary to popular belief, your body is not a 'before' or an 'after'. You do not have to wait in your weight to move your body; by this, I mean you do not need to weigh a certain amount, or look a certain way, to start living a more active life. Fitness is not just reserved for thin people; it can and should be for everyone (as you'll see in the Instagram accounts I've recommended on page 254). As we start to accept our bodies, we stop fighting them and learn to work with them: with respect, kindness, and compassion.

Gentle guidance: Cultivating an intuitive approach to fitness often means taking a necessary break from structure and goals; this is encouraged. As you continue to work on your relationship with fitness, however, you may want to start to set certain goals that you would like to achieve. One example might be running a half-marathon; to do that safely, you will need to add guidance and structure back in. The most important thing is that you should use training plans gently, allowing room for flexibility: give yourself options for extra rest; within your plan, incorporate movement you enjoy; and, ultimately, listen to your body first and the training plan second.

It can be really cool and motivating to have a goal to work towards, but with the principle of gentle guidance, it's no longer about rigid structure but about being able to be flexible in your approach. And you don't have to work towards goals if you don't want to!

Moving beyond health and finding pleasure in moving your body

Jake Gifford MSc
Personal trainer
& PhD student
@ThePhitCoach

Whether it's playing sports at the weekend, riding a bike to and from work, attending a yoga class, or lifting weights as part of a weekly routine, there are many different ways to get our bodies moving. We're frequently told by health professionals and public health campaigns that moving our bodies, whichever way we choose to, is good for our health and something we should be doing more of.[1]

Movement has a long history not only with the promotion of health, but also with anti-fat rhetoric and its associations with moral virtue. More often than not, movement has been a central component to increasingly prevalent weight-loss programmes and lifestyle interventions, which perpetuate the idea that thin bodies are both 'good' and 'healthy' bodies.[2, 3] These narratives often appear in language used by the media and by fitness brands and exercise professionals, where movement is often equated to 'calories burned' and becomes a reflection of our work ethic, something that we 'owe to ourselves and our health'. Consequently the dominant ideas about movement as a primary vehicle for health, 'self-improvement' and weight loss often overshadow forgotten aspects such as pleasure and enjoyment.

Research has highlighted how important pleasure and enjoyment can be in helping us move our bodies over the long term.[4, 5] Pleasure can be experienced in many different ways, including via our senses, through a sense of structure or purpose, or focusing on the activity itself,[6] whether it's hitting a personal best in the swimming pool, the feeling of blood pumping through your body during a workout, or enjoying a walk as part of your daily routine. Pleasure is also connected to our social interactions and the physical spaces where activity takes place, such as outdoors, sports clubs, or gyms. We might get pleasure from the buzz of an energetic class, the serenity of the studio during a gentle yoga flow, or the joy of a bike ride in the sun with friends. Pleasure isn't just about what we do, but where and with whom we do it, too.

If we want to bring pleasure to our activities, we'll need to take a step back and reflect on our relationship with movement. We'll need to ask ourselves why we move, what types of activities we enjoy and at what intensities. We'll also need to explore how the spaces where certain activities take place, such as gyms, studios, or the great outdoors, might impact our relationship with movement, too. In doing so, we can challenge the way we think of what it means to be active and how we'd like to be active. During this reflection you may come to discover that you no longer enjoyed the activities you once used to, and that's absolutely fine. It isn't a moral failure or a loss of willpower if we change our minds about an activity. Neither is it particularly rewarding forcing ourselves to engage in an activity we no longer find pleasure in, no matter how much we are told it's 'good for our health'. So if we aim to be active for the long term rather than just a twelve-week programme, we should really seek to get some enjoyment out of it.

Here are some questions to explore to help you reflect on your relationship with movement.

✖ What do you think about the activity you currently engage in?

✖ How do you feel about the activities you've previously engaged in? Are there any activities you'd like to try in the future?

✖ How does the activity you currently engage in make you feel?

✖ What sensations do you commonly associate with the different activities you've engaged in?

✖ Do you ever feel motivated to engage in a particular activity again?

✖ What do you look forward to when participating in your chosen activity?

✖ What puts you off participating in certain activities?

✖ Would you change the way you get active if enjoyment was the primary reason?

FIGURING OUT MOVEMENT THAT YOU ENJOY

If we've come from a place of relying on punishing workout programmes and fitness trackers to tell us how and when to move our bodies, it can be tricky to know which forms of movement we do actually enjoy! Let's take a closer look at how we can discover finding ways to bring more pleasure to the activities we do and the ways we move our body: start by answering the following questions about the overall experience.

Under the following headings, answer each of the questions to help you figure out what you prefer about the aspects of different activities. There's no right or wrong answer, and you might want to redo this activity periodically to see if things have shifted. The idea is just to help you get more in tune with how you like to move your body, but remember that this may change depending on context, too – for example, a run along the seafront might not be your vibe in the middle of winter, when throwing down your yoga mat and finding a low-key YouTube video could be more your scene.

Environment

____ Do you enjoy getting some fresh air while you're moving your body?

____ Or do you prefer to stay cosy and dry inside?

____ Do you like loud music and bright lights?

____ Do you enjoy spending time around/in water?

____ Do you enjoy spending time in nature when you're moving your body?

Community and connection

Think about whether you like spending time and doing activities on your own or with other people.

_____ Do you enjoy having lots of other people around (like in a class setting)?

_____ Or do you prefer being with just a few friends?

_____ Do you like team games?

_____ Do you prefer doing your own thing in the company of a couple of other people?

_____ Do you enjoy spending time moving your body on your own?

_____ Is it important for you to have a community, for instance a running group, or a group of fat people? For some people movement is also socializing!

Experience

_____ How do you like to feel during and after physical activity?

_____ Do you like feeling strong, focused, energized?

_____ Do you enjoy getting your blood pumping and feeling invigorated?

_____ Or do you like to feel calm and centred?

CONNECTING WITH HOW MOVEMENT MAKES US FEEL

Clients often tell me that they like how movement makes them feel *afterwards*. This reminds me of the diet culture mantra 'no pain, no gain'. And while we can have a bit of an afterglow from movement, if it's not pleasurable at the time, then it's unlikely to be sustainable, or might just feel punishing. Just something to noodle on and notice the subtle ways diet culture can infiltrate our thinking.

Another way of approaching this is trying to connect more with how movement makes us feel in the moment, as well as the lasting impact it has. In clinic I use an *embodied physical activity journal* (see template below) to raise non-judgemental awareness of how much and the type of movement that feels good to us. It also helps us notice our edges and when we need rest.

Before we use the journal though, I often find it helpful to pause and reflect on how it feels when we're not moving much at all; consider this your baseline.

Think of a time where you haven't been able to move much at all – perhaps having to sit at a desk for long periods of time to hit a deadline, or maybe you've been on bed rest recovering from illness or injury.

What were the physical feelings and sensations you experienced?

* Restlessness

* Fidgety

* Slumped shoulders

* Backache

* Like you needed to stretch

* Like you had lots of energy to burn

* Insomnia

* Poor concentration

* ....

What were the emotions and feelings you experienced?

* Frustration

* Anxiety

* Low mood

* Apathy

* ....

Having established a baseline, we can have a clearer idea of the signs and signals our mind and body send when they could benefit from some movement. Now on the flip side, imagine a time when you've been way overdoing it and pushing yourself to the limits with exercise.

What were the physical feelings and sensations you experienced?

* Injuries that took forever to heal

* Stress fractures

* Missing your period

* Long recovery times between training sessions

* More infections and feeling run-down

* Feeling physical symptoms of stress

* ....

What were the emotions and feelings you experienced?

* ✱ Anxiety

* ✱ Stress

* ✱ Guilt

* ✱ Shame

* ✱ Depression

* ✱ ....

Now we've identified how we felt at times where we haven't been able to move as much as we'd like versus periods where we were moving more than was good for our bodies, it can help us find our limits and figure out a way of moving that is supportive and self-caring. In the next activity we'll explore ways of moving that feel supportive and self-caring.

EMBODIED PHYSICAL ACTIVITY JOURNAL

This journal template can help deepen your understanding of how you connect with movement. Use it to check in with how movement feels during an activity; tune into the physical sensations of your muscles, breathing, and exertion. After the activity you might want to consider the less direct physical effects of the activity. Does it help you sleep? Do you feel more alert? How is your mood? In the comments column write down any other observations that you made about the activity. Intuitive movement exists somewhere between these two extremes – a balance between rest and getting your blood pumping. Intuitive movement helps us feel more connected to our bodies, not less.

Some terms to help fill in the table:

Sluggish	Tired	Energized
Stressed	Calm	Motivated
Focused	Unfocused	Achy
Anxious	Depleted	Exhausted
Bored	Exhilarated	Strong
Fidgety	Endorphins	Frustrated
Apathetic	Low mood	Galvanized

Date	Activity	How did you feel . . .? During activity		
		Pleasant	Unpleasant	Neutral

Reflections from the journal activity

Answer the following questions – you can either write them out, or just use them for reflection

* How am I feeling in my body today?

* How does movement or rest influence that?

* Did exercise affect my mood, concentration and energy levels?

* How does movement influence how I feel about my body?

* How did I sleep in the evening afterwards?

* Did this activity help me feel connected to my body?

* Do I have any aches and pains – does exercise help or exacerbate the problem?

How did you feel . . .? After activity					Comments	Did this bring me joy/pleasure
Alertness	Mood	Stress	Sleep	Energy		

+ How can you disconnect movement from diets and diet culture?

+ What does an intuitive relationship with movement look like and feel like for you?

+ How can you tell if you are moving intuitively?

+ Have you noticed any fairy lights switch on?

+ Are there any tools from this section that you can add to your toolkit? Go back to Chapter 1 and write them in.

Listen to the corresponding podcast episode Don't Salt My Game – How to Just Eat It: Chapter 11

CHAPTER 11

GENTLE NUTRITION

Eating disorders can manipulate and distort nutrition information so it's important to follow your team's guidance around a meal plan. However, learning to relax rigid rules, and that nutrition isn't all or nothing, is important. Ask your recovery team for their perspective on this section so you can explore it together.

Merriam Webster defines nutrition as 'the act or process of nourishing or being nourished'. To me this highlights that fundamentally, first and foremost, nutrition is about getting enough to eat. But also that 'being nourished' doesn't just happen on a physical level, but on an emotional one too. As I've said all along, food is greater than the sum of its parts; it's tradition, memories, adventure, grief, culture, family, friendship, love, and everything in between. As long as we see food only as fuel, it will remain something to be optimized, mastered, conquered, and perfected. If you notice yourself approaching food like this, take a step back and try and reframe it as self-care. Gentle nutrition refers to the idea of applying nutrition information in a way that is self-caring, rather than as a tool for self-flagellation. It's about understanding how different foods help you feel and how they help you function. In gentle nutrition, we move away from absolutes (calorie counts, grams of this or that nutrient) and determine what helps us feel well in our bodies. For instance, instead of calculating how many grams of fibre are in each meal, we notice how our digestive health is feeling: are we a bit blocked up and sluggish and in need of some wholegrains? Or are we a little low on energy and want to explore how it feels to add an extra portion of fruit or veg? Likewise, gentle nutrition recognises that if we restrict tasty foods from our diet, then we are likely to obsess about them and then potentially binge on them to compensate for the feelings of deprivation. Gentle nutrition also means including those tasty foods regularly. However, if you are still in the diet mentality of feeling like you have to 'perfect' nutrition, or micromanage every-thing you eat, then you might not yet be ready for gentle nutrition. It might be worthwhile spending some time looking at the quiz in the Introduction to help you identify any areas you might want to revisit before moving on. If you don't feel like nutrition has to be perfect, and you can approach it as a form of self-care, then let's keep on truckin'. I'm not a fan of prescriptive nutrition advice, so you won't find that here, just simple, overarching principles – most of us already know the fundamentals of what constitutes a balanced diet; getting caught up with numbers, grams, portions, and so on can undermine our intuition around food so I won't list them here. However, if you have a concern about nutrition, please speak to a qualified and regulated nutrition professional (preferably one who practices from an intuitive eating perspective!).

THE FOUNDATIONS OF
GENTLE NUTRITION

I hope you're sitting down because I'm going to reveal to you the secrets of a healthy diet. Ready? This might just blow your socks off!

Adequacy Eating regularly and eating enough sound simple, but it's easy to fall back into the diet mentality trap, or to just get busy with life and forget to keep your fuel tank topped up. Erratic eating patterns and insufficient energy can cause problems for immunity, bones, digestion, and hormonal health – among other things. This doesn't have to be rigid, but remember to regularly check in with your hunger cues. Sometimes we need to apply a little logic; if you know it's been a long time between meals and snacks, try and eat something, even if you're not super hungry, and see how you feel.

Balance Lots of trendy diets will try to convince you that you need to cut whole food groups out (see the low-carb trend). This can lead to feelings of physical and emotional deprivation, which backfires as feeling out of control around those foods. Most people need to get a balance of proteins, fats, and carbs. Not necessarily at every meal, but throughout the day. However, if you have, say, a chicken salad for lunch, how does that feel compared to if you were to have some bread or pasta (i.e. carbs) with that chicken salad? You're more likely to have sustained energy, better digestion, and improved mood than without. Without being too rigid about it, I tend to suggest we get some proteins, fats, carbohydrates, dairy (or alternatives), and fibre foods (fruit and veg) most days. We don't need to over-think it or micromanage it.

Variety The best way to ensure that we are meeting our nutritional needs is through getting lots of variety. Rigidly eating the same things day in, day out, means the nutrients we are being exposed to become limited, increasing our chances of deficiency. Eating a wide variety of different flavours, textures, cuisines, and types of food gives us a good chance of hitting our nutrient needs.

Adding in rather than taking away A lot of nutrition advice is grounded in the idea of cutting out 'bad' foods. From a gentle nutrition perspective, we always think about what we can add in rather than take away. For example, if we're feeling a bit blocked up, could we add in some nuts and seeds, wholegrains, or other higher-fibre foods? Or if we are trying to manage blood sugar, instead of cutting out carbs (which could intensify carb cravings), can we add in proteins, fats, and fibre that help keep blood sugar levels more steady after a meal?

Flexibility This means being able to go with the flow. If we're having a super stressful day with no time to cook, can we give ourselves permission to eat toast for dinner? Likewise, if a friend is having a crisis and needs a pizza date stat, can you go and support them sans guilt? Gentle nutrition is knowing that not every meal or snack is 'perfect', but helps us put eating into context. Sometimes it's more important to eat the toast and get yourself to bed rather than staying up late cooking and missing out on sleep. Diet culture teaches us that we are robots who must eat the same number of calories, macros, or points each day. But as life twists and turns, what we eat will shift and change in response.

Self-care Gentle nutrition means nutrition as self-care and doing what you can for yourself, given the limitations of your circumstances. For example, maybe you're a student, stuck in the library during exams; you might not have the capacity to cook a hot meal every night, but can you pack some peanut butter and jam sandwiches to keep your concentration levels topped up? Or maybe you have chronic fatigue; instead of using up the last of your spoons on meal prep, can you keep some ready meals in the freezer? Remember that food can form part of your emotional toolkit, too – sometimes we just need chocolate or ice cream.

> **A note on illnesses:** nutrition is often packaged up as being a way of 'fixing' or 'hacking' a condition. And while it's true that nutrition can help support management of a condition, there aren't many instances where nutrition can 'cure' health concerns altogether. Remember that it's one tool we can use to help and support ourselves, but it's not the be-all and end-all. If you are working on managing a specific health concern, then I recommend getting support from a nutrition professional who specializes in intuitive eating. They will be able to help you navigate your condition with self-compassion and kindness. My clinic also produces some simple guides to managing specific health conditions through an intuitive eating lens – check out gumroad.com/lcie

Just a little word of caution – when we hear about the concepts of balance and variety, we often think 'moderation' follows. But moderation is a sneaky diet culture concept that's subtle code for 'restriction'. Think about it: who has ever told you to eat apples or carrots in moderation? Exactly. It's very easy to turn moderation into a rule, so in the context of gentle nutrition, we bin it.

> Step back and write down what you'd consider to be the basics of a healthy, balanced diet. Don't overthink it.

Choosing what to eat is like getting dressed

Paige Smathers RDN
Nutrition therapist
and host of Nutrition
Matters podcast
@paigesmathersrd

One of the most common questions I get as a dietitian is this: What should I eat?

While I understand why people ask this question, I also struggle to answer it in any kind of straightforward way. There are so many different patterns of eating that nourish and satisfy, and there really isn't a right or wrong way to eat. But there is a fairly simple metaphor that can help to provide a bit of structure while allowing for individualization in deciding what to eat.

Choosing what to eat is a lot like choosing what to wear.

With getting dressed, there's a loose formula: you wear something on top, something on the bottom, and some type of shoe. There are infinite combinations of how this might look, and it all depends on weather, style, mood, and the function I need the clothes to serve. And there are days where I make the call that I'm not putting on shoes, or refuse to wear trousers, and that's totally fine! Wearing a shirt, trousers, and shoes, isn't a *rule*. It's simply a loose formula for getting dressed that works well on most days.

Getting dressed has a lot of similarities with feeding ourselves. It's something we have to do daily, even when we don't want to. Both getting dressed and feeding ourselves affect the way we feel and the way we function. We take many factors into account in getting dressed, but in the end it's guesswork. Eating is guesswork too: there's no perfect. You simply make a guess and move on. And just like there's no right or wrong way to dress yourself, there's no right or wrong way to feed yourself.

Just like there's a loose structure with getting dressed, there's also a loose structure with food: protein, carbohydrate, fat, and fibre at a meal tend to yield the highest likelihood of satisfaction and nourishment. And just like it isn't a rule that you have to wear a shirt, trousers, and shoes daily, it's also not a rule that you have to eat every meal with this formula. There's room for individual preference with food, just like there's room for individual expression with clothing.

Here's how I get dressed: I take a look in my closet and usually something pops out as something that I'd like to wear. My next question is: what else do I want to add to it that will work for my day (taking into account weather, function, my mood, etc)? I also check in with how I feel and how I need these clothes to function for me (i.e. I'll wear something different if I'm going to work versus volunteering in my child's class versus going on a hike).

Food can be similar: take a look at what sounds good (or what's available, convenient) and then ask yourself what you can add to that food to nourish and satisfy you. Do you need to add some bread? Some protein? A fruit or veggie? Some type of dip or fat to help increase the satisfaction of the meal?

You will very likely veer from this formula with food. That's OK! In fact, I'd argue it's healthy and positive to have enough flexibility to be able to veer from this formula. Just like it's fun and positive to have a day where you wear your bathing suit all day at the beach, meals without all the elements of the formula are normal, health-promoting, and OK too.

Notice how it feels to get dressed on days when you feel pressure to wear 'the right thing', for instance days where you're giving a presentation, or going on a first date, or getting ready for an interview for your dream job. Is it harder to get dressed when you feel pressure to be perfect? It's also far harder to feed yourself when you put unnecessary pressure on yourself to do it 'just right'.

You'll likely notice that feeding yourself gets far easier when you let go of the belief that there's a 'right way' to do it. There are infinite iterations of meals that can both nourish and satisfy you. There's room for your individual preferences, personal style, and your unique values to shine through in how you dress yourself, just like there's room for all of that in how you feed yourself.

Questions

✖ How do you typically get dressed? What do you notice about your thought patterns with getting dressed?

✖ Do you notice any similarities between getting dressed and feeding yourself?

✖ Do you notice it's harder to get dressed when you feel pressure to wear just the right thing?

I want to acknowledge that choosing what to wear is not always as simple as I speak about here. I own that I have a lot of privilege in being able to open my closet and choose what to wear in a relatively low-stress way. I recognize that for many this is a highly emotional topic. Finding clothes that fit and having options you feel good in are really important things to consider for a healthy relationship with food. That's another reason this metaphor is powerful.

MENU PLANNING

Menu planning is *not* essential – sometimes the mental burden of making shopping lists and figuring out what your week is going to look like is just *too much*. I get that, and for you I've included a quick shopping list to get you by later on in this section. However, clients often say to me that they want a little guidance on how to approach menu planning from an intuitive eating perspective, without falling back into diet mentality or 'meal prep' mode.

Step 1 Before you get started, here are some things to consider.

* Check in with your intention behind menu planning – is it coming from a place of self-care? Or self-control and fear?

* It can be helpful to reframe this as your 'menu' for the week – not as a 'plan' that you have to stick to rigidly. Remember to consider which days/meals you may be eating out or if you have to pick something up.

* Think about balancing your meals – this isn't a hard and fast, but a little gentle nutrition guidance to help you cover all your bases: grains, protein, fibre, fat, and dairy/dairy alternatives. Don't worry if you don't check all the boxes at each meal or snack, just notice how it feels. For instance, how are your mood and energy levels when you skip the grains at lunch? Is the rest of the afternoon a total slog?

* Don't forget a fun food – meals are something to look forward to and enjoy.

* Think about playing with flavours, textures, and temperatures, and get plenty of variety where you can. Think about which type of cuisine you might want to experiment with, and consider adding a new recipe to your repertoire.

* Look for inspiration from your favourite chefs, home cooks, and recipe books, rather than from 'clean eaters', which can leave you feeling unsatisfied. It can be worth bookmarking some of your favourite recipes to come back to when planning your menu.

* I always recommend including quick and easy options for those days that you won't have the time or the energy to cook from scratch – ready meals in the freezer are a great option so you don't always end up having toast for dinner. A ready-made pizza with a salad is another. And don't forget the humble beans on toast with cheese on top – economical, quick, balanced, and satisfying.

* Give yourself permission to be flexible – if your friend calls you up and asks you for a last-minute dinner date (assuming you want to go), can you shuffle things about a bit? Remember, ultimately intuitive eating is about being flexible, so you don't miss out on other important aspects of your life that dieting often steals from you.

* Remember that your menu is about being kind to yourself, not something to beat yourself up about if things don't go to plan. Be gentle with yourself if your week gets turned on its head and you end up working late and eating a takeaway at the office. That curry you batch-cooked can be thrown in the freezer to stop it going off.

* Don't forget to schedule in some self-care each day – it can be low-key, like going for a walk or listening to a podcast, or boring but important stuff like doing laundry, going to the doctor or therapy, or simply just resting.

Copy these questions out into your journal to help you plan for the week

Step 2 Here are some questions that might be helpful for you when planning your menu for the week. These help you focus on aspects of the meal aside from the minutiae of points, calories, or other diet-y distractions. But I get that it's a lot to think about this every week. It might be worth doing it a few times until you get familiar with the types of things that are most important to you, and then narrowing down your shortlist of things to consider when menu planning.

Menu for the week of _____

* How's the weather looking this week? Do I want hot/cold options? Do I want something warming or cooling or a mixture of options?

* Which flavours and textures am I craving? Salty, spicy, sweet, umami, creamy, crunchy, gooey, flaky, wholesome, comforting, refreshing?

* How's my energy level and time availability this week? Do I want to cook from scratch or do I need some more convenient options?

* Which days am I busy and need to pick something up on the go or have plans to go out to eat? When might I want a packed lunch?

* Is there any specific food I've been craving that I could add into my rotation this week? (i.e. a bowl of cheesy pasta)

* Can I double up any of my recipes to stick in the freezer or have as leftovers?

* Breakfast ideas for this week:

....

＊ Snack ideas for this week:

....

＊ Main meal ideas for this week:

....

＊ Fun food and dessert ideas for this week:

....

＊ A new meal, dish, or snack I want to try:

....

Step 3 Fill out as much or as little of the menu table as feels good to you.

	Monday	Tuesday	Wednesday	Thursday	Friday	Saturday	Sunday
Breakfast							
Snack							
Lunch							
Snack							
Dinner							
Snack							
Self-care activity for today							

Quick shopping checklist

Eliza Khinsoe, RD
Nutrition counsellor at the London Centre for Intuitive Eating and host of The Pantry Party podcast
@lizakhins
@thepantryparty

For most of my life, I've lived in suburban Australia, where supermarkets are gigantic but few and far between. It's typical there for one member of the household to do a big weekly or fortnightly shop, driving the fifteen minutes to the supermarket to get everything you need. This would then be supplemented by weekend trips to farmers' markets, or quick trips to the corner shop when you've run out of milk. (Obviously, I can't speak for all Australians: the way we access our food varies hugely by location, family dynamics, culture, food preferences, you name it, and my own experience was one with a great deal of privilege, as it involved having the time, money, food knowledge, and access to a car.)

So when I moved to London, the food environment here had me SHOOK. There's a supermarket on every corner, and dozens of convenience stores, corner shops, and greengrocers that make it easy to grab food on the go. To my dismay, I found that it's not feasible to have a giant, fully stocked pantry and fridge – and people here tend to work longer hours and use public transport, so it's difficult to find the time or the arm strength to shop for a week's worth of food at a time.

I had to learn how to relax my meal plans throughout the week, adapt to having access to ready meals (which are totally not a thing Down Under), and let go of my structure, routine, and neat weekly menu plan, in favour of a more flexible eating pattern that would fit around my new lifestyle. One of the most valuable things I learned was how to pop into the supermarket on my way home from work, and so I'm going to share that with you.

So, let's set the scene. It's 6pm on a Tuesday night, you're on your way home and are exhausted from a busy day. As you're contemplating the evening ahead of you, two things flicker into your awareness. The first is that you're hungry – all the work you've done in bringing attention to your hunger throughout this book has come in handy, and your body's sending you a loud and clear signal that it's time to eat! The second thing is that dreadful sinking realization that currently the only residents of your fridge are a jar of mustard and half a sad-looking cabbage. You could order a pizza, but you also need milk for your breakfast and some lunch for tomorrow, so you decide to stop by the shop.

Now here's the tricky part. When we're hungry, our executive functioning often goes out the window in favour of a primal feeling of 'NEED FOOD NOW', so it can be difficult to think about planning, complex recipes, or that thing you keep meaning to add to your shopping list. But I'm assuming you're not standing at the entrance of the supermarket reading this, so we've got a little time to do that now.

My first tip is to keep a running shopping list on your phone, so it's with you wherever you go. Get into the habit of using it, and if you shop for other people, share it with them so they can add to it too.

Next, come up with a few go-to, super simple meals that you enjoy. Things like pasta with a pre-made sauce and frozen veg, an omelette with cheese and toast, jazzed-up instant noodles (add some veg and an egg and you're good to go), your favourite ready meals, or a stir-fry kit. Make a note of them and keep that on your phone, too. That way, when you're waiting for the train and your hunger hits, you can peruse it like a menu and see if anything takes your fancy.

Then do a quick scan over what you know you've usually got at home and think about the next couple of days and the foods you enjoy.

Now copy the template below into your journal to create your go-to quick shopping list

✔	Category	Example	Your turn
	1 Ready meal/ convenience food	Pasta ready meal	
	2 Grains	Bagels, rice	
	3 Protein/dairy foods	Tin of chickpeas, cream cheese, milk	
	4 Fruit and veg (fresh/ tinned/frozen)	Carrots, spinach, apples, frozen broccoli	
	5 Fun foods, flavour, snacks & sauces	Bag of nuts, orange juice, curry sauce, ice cream, pack of cookies	

Remember: it doesn't have to be perfect, and it's OK to have boring, convenient, and bland foods sometimes. But try to go for foods you enjoy, rather than the things diet culture says you should be eating.

+ Does your shopping style suit your lifestyle? How can you make it easier for yourself?

+ What are your beliefs about convenience foods? Are they justified?

+ Are you able to offer yourself compassion around shopping for quick, easy, and tasty foods?

MAKING PEACE WITH ALL FOODS

At this stage in the game, I'm hoping that you've really embraced the idea of no good foods or bad foods, and are leaning into the concept of food neutrality. That's not to say there aren't foods that might make us feel better or function better – but that doesn't mean they're good or bad, just that they 'work' for our bodies. But there may still be some resistance to eating these foods – they may be foods you associate with dieting, deprivation, restriction, 'clean' eating, or 'being good' in the past. It's understandable that we may want to rebel against this. So how can we reconcile the fact that there are foods we might want to eat more of because they make us feel good, without pulling ourselves back into diet mentality? You might have already figured this out from some of the activities earlier in the book (check you out!), but finding pleasure in these foods is HUGE. We've focused a lot on making peace with foods we might have once considered 'bad', but we might also need to consider making peace with foods we once thought of as 'good'. We can also bring a sense of curiosity and non-judgement to these foods – do they really not taste good to me, or has my perception been distorted because we are taught vegetables (for instance) are gross? How do I feel when I incorporate more higher-fibre foods into my diet? How's my energy, digestion, and sense of well-being? How can I make nutritious foods more enjoyable and pleasurable?

Here are some ideas you might like to consider:

* Roasting vegetables in oil or topping with butter (fats help us absorb more nutrients from veg anyway, so why wouldn't you?).

* Trying new ways to incorporate beans – adding kidney beans to chilli, cooking refried black beans for Taco Tuesday, making your own super creamy hummus with chickpeas (or go rogue

and make different types of bean dips), test out different bean burgers available in your local supermarket (rank them to make it more fun). But also, a good old can of Heinz counts as one of your 5-a-day – add toast and cheese and you have one of the most wholesome of meals ever conceived.

* Play with salad dressings – no one wants to eat naked salad, so dress that puppy up, and add loads of fun elements too. Salads don't need to be boring!

* Don't forget that fruit and veg don't need to be complicated. If the resistance for you was that they need a lot of prep – peeling, chopping, long cooking times – remember that this is exactly why frozen versions exist. Peas, sweetcorn, and carrots from a bag 'count' just as much as fresh. Ditto dried and canned. You can also get stir-fry mixes and other medleys.

* Frozen fruit thrown into a blender with milk or yoghurt is all you need for a refreshing smoothie – you don't need fancy superfood blends or protein powders – although adding a generous amount of peanut butter or oats might help make them more satisfying and filling. Equally juice or smoothie from a carton might be more your bag.

* Try experimenting with cooking grains in different ways – quinoa and brown rice can be pretty dull on their own, so what can you do to jazz them up?

* ....
Add your own ideas here, too

* ....

* ....

* ....

In your journal, make a note of the answers to the following questions

What are some nutritious foods you associate with dieting or restriction that you might rebel against eating?

Are there any of these foods that you'd like to have a better relationship with?

What can you do to cast off the diet-y association and make them more appealing?

Can you tap into how these foods make you feel in your body, as well as how they taste?

+ Can you notice how food feels in your body as a whole – mouth, digestive system, in terms of energy, mood, and overall sense of well-being?

+ Are your eating choices becoming more flexible?

+ What are some meals or snacks that leave you feeling both content/satisfied and nourished?

+ Have any more fairy lights switched on for you?

+ Are there any tools in this section that you can add to your toolkit? Go back to Chapter 1 and write them in.

CHAPTER 12
WHERE WE GO FROM HERE

Intuitive eating is a means to an end; it's a set of tools to liberate us from the clutches of food rules and body hatred. Intuitive eating gives us freedom from diet culture: freedom to focus on things that are bigger and more important to us. Maybe they are personal ambitions, like starting our own business, or going back to school or studies. Or maybe they're bigger picture issues, like engaging more in our community, getting political, or advocating for social justice issues. Connecting with these things can bring a sense of purpose and fulfilment based on internal contentment, rather than the external validation that diet culture perpetuates.

In this section I want to help you start to explore some bigger picture issues through the lens of intuitive eating. We'll explore race, disability, and poverty. Through a series of guest essays, we'll consider the privilege that is an inherent part of being able to eat intuitively. While intuitive eating is the default for many of us as children, there are structural, political, and physical barriers that prevent people from accessing the full expression of intuitive eating. It's important to acknowledge that while diet culture is a system of oppression in and of itself, it's not working in isolation. For many people, the impact is confounded by identities that are marginalized in society.

I also want you to consider what's next for you. We'll take a fresh look at the brain activity you did right at the very beginning, so you can reflect on 'what's next', as well as check in with your values.

By now, I hope you are feeling a lot more comfortable with the practice of intuitive eating and are heading towards the 'what's the big deal?' phase (see Introduction, page 25) – although if you're not there yet, that's cool too. You can take a look back at the intuitive eating quiz on page 26 to get some clues as to which areas it would be good to have another look at. If you feel like you're pretty much getting it, then it's reasonable to think 'what's next?' Diets keep us stuck in a perpetual loop of falling on and off the 'bandwagon', whereas my hope for intuitive eating is that it integrates into your life and allows you to practice flexibility, so there is no bandwagon to fall off. This means we have the freedom and headspace to lead a meaningful life outside of diet culture. That's what we'll explore here.

Checking in with our values

One way of answering the 'what's next?' question is to reflect back on the values assessment you did in Chapter 1. Flip back to the bullseye on page 65, and remind yourself:

* How aligned or unaligned were you with particular values in different domains of life?

* Which values or domains were you hoping to dedicate more time/space/energy to?

Now, let's revisit the bullseye. Using the blank template on page 309, fill it out for each of your core values. Think about where you're at *currently*, after having done some work on intuitive eating.

Remember, for the domains in which you feel you align with your values the most, you'll mark towards the centre of the bullseye. Next, go to your journal and answer the following:

*   Compared to before you embarked on the intuitive eating process, do you feel you are more aligned with your values in some areas? Which?

*   Are there any areas in which you'd like to be guided more by your values?

*   Are your core values the same as when you began this process, or have your priorities changed at all?

*   Does this help provide clarity about what lies beyond intuitive eating for you? In other words, which values-driven goals do you have for yourself?

If you're ever feeling lost or stuck, and are starting to notice those diet-y thoughts coming back in, return to this activity to help refocus on what's most important in helping you live a fulfilling, values-driven life.

How you fill your headspace

In Chapter 2, we spent some time reflecting on how much head-space is taken up by thoughts of dieting, nutrition, exercising, and changing your body – and how you'd like to spend that headspace instead. Now's a good time to check in and see how much band-width you're dedicating to the activities you enjoy, versus the ones diet culture dictates you 'should' do. This isn't to say that a portion of your headspace shouldn't be taken up by gentle nutrition and intuitive movement (if those things are important to you); it's more that they should take up an appropriate amount of space, so that we're not overthinking them. That way, our mental energy isn't skewed towards them, so we have energy to focus on all the things that are important to us.

Refer back to the brain activity you completed on page 83 that depicted how you'd like your headspace to be filled as an intuitive eater.

* How does your actual brain compare to the drawings you did on pages 82 and 83? Does it more closely resemble the 'intuitive eating' brain or the 'diet' brain?

* How are you spending the extra headspace freed up by ditching diet culture?

* Are there activities, goals, interests, or hobbies that you want to pursue now you've ditched diet culture?

THINKING BEYOND OUR OWN PERSONAL INTUITIVE EATING PROCESS

Intuitive eating is often portrayed as a solo endeavour, which can divorce it from the bigger picture and distract us from how much of a privilege it is to renounce diet culture. In the following essays, three guest contributors explore the ways in which intuitive eating may be inaccessible to them, to varying degrees. As we contemplate the ways that intuitive eating may, for some of us, have opened up new ways of thinking and experiencing the world, we must also acknowledge that without deeper social justice work, intuitive eating (or elements of it) remains out of reach for so many who are experiencing marginalization. After reading each of the guest essays, be sure to carefully consider the reflection questions that follow.

Imogen Fox, disability rights activist
@the_feeding_of_the_fox

I have lived most of my adult life with some form of restriction around food. As a Disabled person, I've lived in poverty; I've gone without adequate physical support to make food; I've endured disordered eating; and I continue to have a condition that makes eating, digesting, and absorbing food almost impossible.

When I entered the world of intuitive eating and body liberation, I felt very strongly the desire to be part of such a political and radical movement. Having spent so much of my life fighting for the rights of Disabled people, but still feeling desperate to assimilate to beauty standards, I remember the light bulb moment when I realized it was all inextricably linked. It wasn't much of a shock, though, when I realized how few people like me existed within the movement. Conversations around intuitive eating rarely consider those within intersections, the people in the margins: those of us who already live with the additional pressures that are placed upon us by our social status. Our need to assimilate, for our own safety, when our bodies, class, or financial situation identifies us as divergent — a need that just doesn't exist within privileged communities.

I have lost count of the number of ways I have been denied access to food. Financial hardship; not receiving enough physical support to shop, prepare, or eat meals; undiagnosed/untreated eating disorders or impairments that make eating, digesting, or absorbing food hard or impossible — these only just scratch the surface of the deprivation I've faced when it came to having and eating food.

When you live without wellness in the way that I have, it becomes an elusive status that you're pressed to chase and maintain. When society decides we're not working hard enough

to do so, we are shamed. This feels like a reframe from historical pressures to be 'thin', the focus having shifted to living an
active 'on the go' lifestyle coupled with clean eating. We as a
community are left not only with the lingering societal push to
be healthy, to be 'thin', but also with the additional pressure
of medicine. We are surrounded by seemingly well-meaning,
well-educated healthcare professionals who dole out fat phobia
guised as medical advice. Weight-loss and miracle diets are
dropped into medical appointments and coffee mornings alike;
everyone knows someone who cured your situation with a raw
juice diet, after all.

Wellness culture compels us to believe that food is always
poison and cure. An all or nothing that comes with hard and fast
rules about what you can or can't eat for the sake of yourself. In
my case, each choice I made filled me not only with the weight
of my physical self, but also with the possible impact on my body
and, in turn, my access to medical care.

The things that I hear in my head today aren't my own. Although
we share a voice, they're the words of a thousand different
people who shared a million different opinions over decades
of medical and societal trauma. They're the documentaries on
Netflix, the magazines in the newsagents, the pamphlets in my
GP surgery. Worse still, they're the misguided passing comments
of family, the unsolicited medical advice, and the preachy
Instagram captions of people who 'used' to be just like me but
found the holy grail.

Also vying for space within all of that rhetoric are the practical
scars and stark truths that I have to consider, alongside the
above, every time I contemplate food. Things like my energy
levels, if I have PA/care support, if I'm out in public or near a
toilet. If I'm already in pain, how I've felt the last few hours, where
my headspace is, or if I'm with people who 'get it'.

And through all of this sounds the siren of scarcity. What if there just won't be any more food?

Disabled people, people with long-term health conditions, those of us who will have to interact with medics for possibly the rest of our lives: we are left in static, with no ability to tune into our bodies and respond intuitively to them. We will continue to be weighed at hospital appointments, denied treatment when our bodies are considered too big, or scolded by health practitioners who tut as we attempt to shrink down all the complexities of our everyday into bite-sized chunks they might understand. Our life support is entirely hinged on our ability to 'manage' our bodies to the satisfaction of these gatekeepers, who have the fundamental power to decide if we are worthy of treatment or not.

While the IE community is slowly opening its eyes to the swathes of people who've never been afforded meaningful or safe connection with our bodies, we still fall so far short. How am I meant to have faith in a body that has never been reliable? How am I meant to tune into or trust voices that are fuelled by the harm inflicted on me? How am I meant to grant myself unconditional permission to do anything, when every moment of my life is conditional on my body's ability to function?

When prioritizing 'healthful' choices, what key values are you focusing on? Consider if they are related to thinness or altering your body to meet societal views of 'health', rather than individual needs.

Have you ever had a period of time when you couldn't always choose foods you craved due to medication, short-term illness, or allergies? How did that impact you, your food choices, or your mental health?

When thinking about health, consider mental health, too. If you're making choices, how often do you focus on the mental health implications of the decision you're making?

Could you put in place some firmer boundaries for when you interact with medics in future?

Branavie Ranjithakumaran, BNutSc,
MDiet, non-diet dietitian and public health researcher
@arebrandedlife
@thepantryparty

The world of intuitive eating is trapped behind barriers. At the time of writing, it is 2020, and IE has been co-opted by diet culture, is locked away due to financial restraints, and feels as though it is in a glass case that requires time, emotional capacity, and social support to effect its positive change in the world. As a practitioner and a public health researcher, sometimes I struggle with how out of alignment intuitive eating can be with the social justice principles of Health at Every Size (HAES).

In its simplest form, HAES aims to encourage health promotion behaviours that are independent of body weight, race, gender, class, and other forms of systemic oppression. It addresses the way health lies on a continuum and varies according to each individual, and that each person's capacity to address their health is neither an outcome nor an objective of living. IE therefore supports this, as it provides guidance against the instructive model of health, teaching individuals to be flexible with nutrient intake, while understanding the societal barriers that prevent you from achieving your optimum health.

Both professionally and personally, I have found that those from diverse cultural backgrounds are the ones who are most repelled by the idea of intuitive eating. Intuitive eating requires introspection, reflection, and an acknowledgement to rely on your body instead of objective measures. In summary, it's hard work — it goes against the grain, de-expertises experts, and allows the individual to view what health means to them, as opposed to external validation. Furthermore, the stigma of intuitive eating therapy within these cultures is similar to that of psychological therapy. In the Western world, psychological therapy has, for the most part, made leaps and bounds in the reduction of its stigma. It's accepted, even if people don't overtly encourage the concept. In the Asian world, however, therapy insinuates that you're not strong enough, that you don't have self-control. Asking for help is seen as asking for the destruction of reputation and privacy for families.

Those who have migrated from a non-dominant culture into the Western world feel pressure to 'fit in' to a society that is incredibly critical. Part of this Western assimilation includes the adoption of Western body and health ideals in order not to stand out, and to make life easier for themselves. Those from nations colonized by the Western world often already have these ideals ingrained. To take myself as an example: hailing from a Sri Lankan background, I had a childhood littered with such notions as 'fairer is better' and being praised for my 'slim body' – despite the fact that, genetically, the likelihood of me maintaining this figure for the rest of my life was, as with all bodies, very low.

These slight comments had far more impact than those saying them could have known. They forced me to take on the notion that food from my cultural roots is unhealthy, fattening, glutton-ous, and only reserved for special occasions. I began to distance myself from all things cultural in order to assimilate fully into the Western world, to be seen as successful – successfully shedding my nationality in the process. I'm still repairing these dissoci-ations. I'm ashamed of how quickly I left the principles of my motherland behind, assuming that the Western way of living was better, whether in terms of education, societal values, or body image ideals. For a period of time, the beauty of cultural diver-sity was lost on me, all for the sake of 'health' and 'fitting in'. I'm slowly learning the importance of food in cultural settings as part of IE: the identity, belonging, connection that food gives me – to my cultural heritage, family, and more. This process of connection with food allows me to share deep-rooted cultural notions with the people around me – I can see the joy that people feel when they get a glimpse into food that is delicious, made with love, and socially connective.

Bran's essay explores the nuances of intuitive eating: how it's not just the hunger–fullness diet, and how the science behind health is not diversely determined, so not all cultures are represented in health – for many, resulting in the forced decision to shed the heritage that they come from.

Aside from potentially losing connection to culture through food, how else does the Westernized version of health limit your ability to appreciate your body?

Does it affect how you view your body?

Do you forget or try and dismiss the genetic components of health that you have minimal control over?

Are you given time and space to appreciate what your ancestors have gone through for you to arrive to the body you have?

How can IE help you reconnect with your cultural heritage?

Scottee, artist and broadcaster
@scotteeisfat

Well-meaning therapists, doctors, friends, and followers have
all tried their best to convince me that intuitive eating might
be worth a shot – offering up the answers I'm supposed to be
seeking to address my relationship to my long-reigning agitator.

IE has a cult following – one that is rapidly growing, a mass with
such conviction – often handed over to an invisible power, not
to mention some believers who consider me to be broken until I
see the light. So it's really hard for me, as a recovering Catholic,
to distance their faith in it with my fear of faith.

'You just eat what your body is telling you to eat,' they say, with
ease, as if they know and understand the voice their body has,
its accent and intonation. What they often don't realize is that I
and others like me have never heard our bodies – and we're
likely never going to either, because our bodies don't talk, they
shout, worry, fear.

If my body was a thing, it would be a dodgy KitchenAid rip-off
from the market, constantly churning a dough of feelings not yet
baked. Kneaded and beaten together: shame, guilt, rebellion,
pride, and inadequacy. These would be proved and allowed to
bloat with queerness, fatness, and of course, class.

I say 'of course' because class – being common, having survived
poverty – has informed most, if not all, of me and my immediate
family's relationship with food, and with eating as well. I think the
distinction between food and eating here is important: not only
do I live with compulsion, addiction, and fear of food, but I also
have the noise of eating to contend with, too.

Like many working-class kids, I have a long history with hoarding
food: making sandwiches with cheap white bread, squeezed into

empty takeaway boxes under my bed until they went mouldy. This was largely through fear of scarcity. Fat, common kids like me are now effigies for middle-class woke parents, who blame the parents for not feeding them carrots. We shame working-class and poor families (the differentiation between working class and poor is important here) with food – policing, taxing, depriving – and that shame is transposed, and leaves its mark like a cheap tattoo transfer you used to get with bubblegum in the 1990s. We also think the solution to this is food banks – I wonder how many of us with turbulent relationships with food feel at ease with giving it away? I wonder how many of us who know scarcity are held back from giving to food banks through fear of returning there? I wonder how much of our relationship with food has been informed by free school meals and no-brand cola?

Our history with food and class is long. I come from a working-class Irish migrant family. A family that left the island because of hunger and famine. A family that returned home and left because of poverty, and returned and left again because of poverty. I am the fifth generation to be economically displaced. My feet are now firmer on the ground, and so I hope to be the last, but that trauma is deep: experienced, socialized, historical, and I believe genetic, it's in us to the backbone.

Food has never been about eating in my family. Men eat at the table, women stand. Food is often only functional, to keep you going, but it is also your closest friend. If you've experienced poverty you understand the small amount of softness foods can offer – they are reliable, the one semi-constant. Chocolate, crispy pancakes, and fizzy pop offer solace at accessible prices in a world that is volatile. In the same breath, food was and is a weapon and a tool: for care, repair, healing, and self-flagellation.

So, when I'm asked to respond to what my body wants, to listen to my so-called intuition, what happens is a string of

HOW TO JUST EAT IT

conversations I often don't have the energy to deal with. Take what you can, do what you must, do it quickly before it goes, don't be seen, feel guilty, have an argument with yourself, accept the thoughts, don't panic, you know what this is about, I'm not allowed it, it's against the rules, I don't deserve it . . . the list goes on. Choosing a sandwich for lunch can take the best part of twenty minutes for me, as I let them argue it out in the silent war in my head until someone gives in.

Intuition when you've lived a life that isn't afforded luxury or radical generosity is often a panicked, loaded emotion, and not a gut feeling that can be heard clearly. It is swamped by the cacophony of shame and scarcity, a sound that is often more derailing than living with 'the rules' IE often distances itself from. Survival and managing precariousness take precedence. They become ingrained behaviours, and the roots of our trauma and behaviours need careful unpicking, work that takes more from us than just asking 'Does my body want broccoli today?' We know what we want, we just don't have access to it.

The truth is, I am envious of those who can hear their body and what it has to say, those who have enough clarity to learn its sound. I feel IE often works for those who are able to reach what they want, when they want it, and who have the privilege of asking themselves what it is they want. My therapist recently noted that my relationship to self-care is similarly classed; like IE, I consider it to be a pastime and joy for people who don't sound like me, who are not like me – an experience for those who can afford to be kinder to themselves.

My aim isn't to park with you, but for us to acknowledge class on our messy table of eating. With this in mind, my parting question to you is this: How has class informed your relationship to eating, food, and your body?

Scottee's essay highlights how intuitive eating is not accessible to everyone and that there are structural and sociopolitical barriers that prevent people being able to connect with their bodies.

What other barriers can you think of that might interfere with people being able to eat intuitively?

How can we challenge our expectations of what intuitive eating looks like and means to us, given these barriers?

Do Scottee's experiences resonate with your own?

Are there ways we can address these structural barriers to make intuitive eating more accessible and inclusive to more people?

In our final guest contribution, Eliza from the London Centre for Intuitive Eating team is inviting us to contemplate a question that so many of our clients constantly ask themselves – what will people think?

When we really stop to think about it, tapping into what feels good in our bodies isn't a particularly radical idea, yet it's still so counter-cultural to eat what tastes and feels good, and to let our bodies find their natural setpoint weight, rather than live up to unrealistic beauty ideals. We can spend a lot of time wondering and worrying about what other people think. In this essay and the questions that follow, Eliza invites us to let go of other people's expectations.

What will people think?

Ditching the diets and learning to eat intuitively can be a really liberating process, but for most of us, it's a stepping stone that helps us find body acceptance and food freedom so we can move on to bigger and better things, living our lives the way that we want to. But while this sounds good in theory, putting these ideas into practice can be a whole other ball game.

I exist on the intersections of a bunch of different identities and have spent a lot of time grappling with where I fit in within our society's standards. In the past, I have allowed the fear of what other people will think to hold me back from living my life the way I want to, from being my most authentic self. What will my family think? My friends? Strangers on the street? What might they think about my body? My weight? The way I'm acting, or expressing myself?

It makes sense; the society we live in is built on racist, fat-phobic, heteronormative, and patriarchal standards. We live in fear of judgement and discrimination, which keeps diverse and marginalized people oppressed, and amplifies the power held by the oppressor. But change is happening. We wouldn't be here talking about intuitive eating without the people who fought for equal rights, for acceptance and liberation from these outdated norms. I believe it's our duty to continue this work, and every step we take in solidarity or allyship continues this momentum towards justice.

One way to play your part is to be radically and authentically you, however you identify. To show up, represent, and have pride in who you are. Can you imagine how you'd feel if you saw people like yourself in art, on social media, or out on the streets? How much more time, energy and capacity you would've had if you'd never been taught to hate yourself? Representation is the

Eliza Khinsoe, RD
Nutrition counsellor at the London Centre for Intuitive Eating and host of The Pantry Party podcast
@lizakhins
@thepantryparty

first step in liberation, so if we can show up for ourselves, we're paving the way for others to do so too, making a safer, more inclusive world for everyone.

Showing up for ourselves isn't easy. It takes a conscious decision to be courageous and to choose this consistently over time. It takes work, and it can be scary and exhausting. But the more we do it, the more resilient we become – and the easier it gets. So I wrote this piece as a reminder, for myself and for you, to show up for ourselves when we're worried about what others will think.

What will other people think?

Yes, what will they think?
What do they think when they see you now?
Doing the things you do to adhere to the rules.

Controlling yourself, your body, your voice.
Punishing yourself, shrinking yourself,
diminishing yourself.

What will other people think
when they learn to understand
that that's the only way to be?

That in order to be worthy,
acceptable and successful,
they have to be palatable and subdued.

What will they think about themselves?
Their own body?
Their own voice?
So then, what will other people think
when they see you in all your glory?
Taking up space, showing up, existing?

Leading by example of how to
have a body in this world without
falling victim to these rules?

Modelling behaviour that says
you don't have to change?
You don't have to control yourself.
You don't have to force yourself to fit in,
you don't have to punish yourself,
shrink yourself, diminish yourself.

What will people think
when you show them that
you can exist without hating yourself?

Without having to hold yourself to a set of rules
and expectations that only exist to
keep us small, to keep us quiet.

Exist in this world in a way you wish others had before you.
The people who came before couldn't,
but they suffered for us to have this opportunity.

Use your privilege
and the safety that comes with it
to pave the way for those without.

Break the rules. Show up. Represent.
Use your voice. Celebrate.
Because what will people think?

Read back through this poem, answering the questions it asks in your journal.

What would it look like to exist in all your glory? What would it feel like?

What can you do to work towards that feeling? Set some simple intentions to remind yourself of your commitment to food freedom and body compassion as you move through the world.

Diet culture makes us believe that we have absolute control over our bodies, that we are able to mould and shape them into whichever aesthetic is trending at that moment. We are taught that with enough willpower and determination, we can achieve the 'perfect' body. But the pursuit of patriarchal beauty standards keeps us caught in a battle with our bodies; we become distrusting of them and instead seek out external rules to keep them 'in check'. The constant monitoring, micromanaging, and surveilling of food, exercise, and our bodies is *completely exhausting.* It robs us of time, money, energy, and other precious resources. Diet culture thrives on our insecurities and vulnerabilities. It takes advantage of and profits from feelings of low self-worth – which it has manufactured in the first place. Stepping outside of diet culture, saying 'fuck you' to its regressive, anti-feminist agenda, takes gall, strength, and determination. So, if you've made it this far, you're a rock star. It's not easy to go against the grain and stand up for yourself. It's even harder to fight for a fairer, more just world in which all bodies, and I mean ALL bodies, are respected. Black, trans, disabled bodies. Fat bodies, poor bodies, older bodies, and all the bodies who are made to feel anything less than worthy, whom society treats cruelly and unjustly. Intuitive eating may start as a tool for liberating us from diet culture and helping us heal our relationship with food and our bodies, but

I hope that it leads you to fight for body liberation for all. In the resources that follow, you'll find books, podcasts, and activists that can help deepen your learning and find opportunities to take action.

On a personal level, I hope this book has helped you find more peace, and freedom to exist in your body without shame. I hope it has helped bring more joy and pleasure from the foods you eat. I hope it has helped you redefine what health means for you. And I hope it has helped you tap into and trust your internal wisdom, instinct, and intuition.

APPENDIX

EXTRA BITS

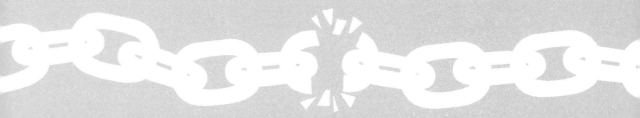

BLANK VALUES BULLSEYE

The following template is to help you check in with your values and notice where you are most closely aligned and where you may want to put more attention. Make as many copies as you might like of the blank template and stick it in your journal. Look back at pages 64–6 for full instructions on how to complete the bullseye.

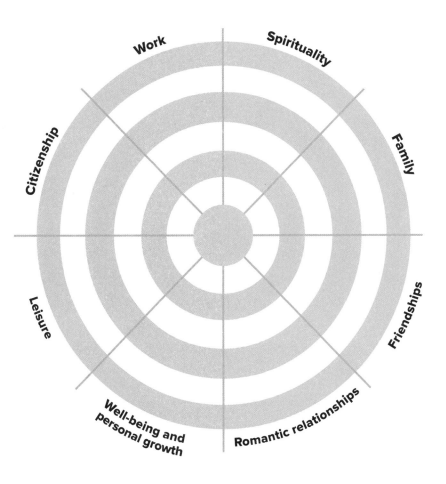

HUNGER AND SATISFACTION GUIDE

Carefully cut along the dotted line around your hunger and satisfaction guide. Cut out a similar-sized piece of card (e.g. from an old cereal packet) and glue the guide on top. Do the same for the arrow. Carefully pierce the dot on the arrow and the dot on the guide with scissors, then securely fasten the two together with a butterfly clip or split pin. You can annotate your guide with what each point along the wheel feels like for you using the word bank.

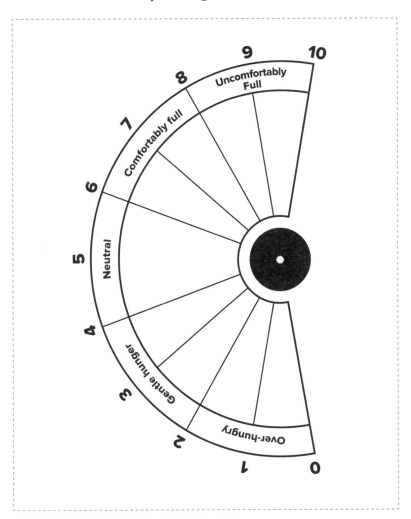

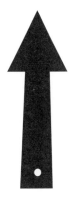

Comfortably full	Neither hungry nor full
Content	Neutral
Cranky	Sense of wellbeing
Distracted	Shaky
Eating slows down	Stomach ache
Empty	Stomach growling
Hangry	Stuffed
Happy	Thinking about food
Headache	Unsatisfied
Hunger pangs	Weak
Light-headed	
Nausea	

FOOD ICONS

Cut out the following food shapes – you will use these for various different activities throughout the book, so you might want to keep them safe in an envelope. If you're really fancy you might even like to laminate them! It's up to you whether or not you colour them in, but it could be a fun mindful colouring project. Alternatively, you could cut out and use food pictures from old magazines or newspapers.

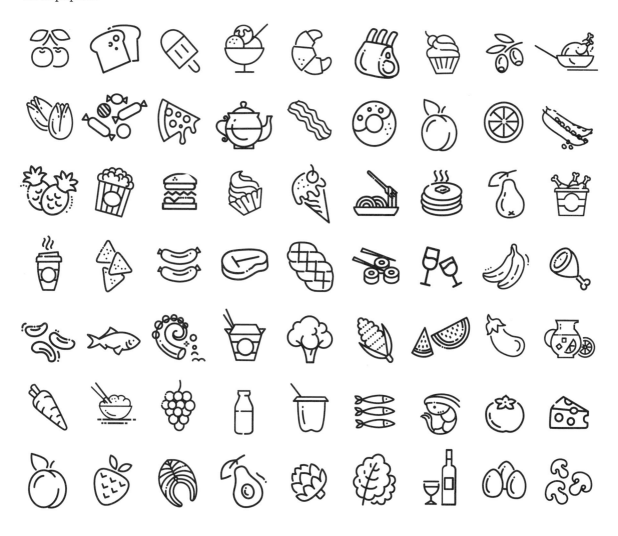

INTUITIVE EATING JOURNAL TEMPLATE

The following template isn't intended to be used as a 'food diary', but as a tool to help you connect with and reflect on your experiences with food. Notice when your automatic mind chimes in with critical thoughts versus when your observer mind makes connections without passing judgement.

Meal/snack:	Meal/snack:	Meal/snack:	Meal/snack:	Meal/snack:	Meal/snack:
How long since I last ate:	How long since I last ate:	How long since I last ate:	How long since I last ate:	How long since I last ate:	How long since I last ate:
What I ate:	What I ate:	What I ate:	What I ate:	What I ate:	What I ate:
How I'm feeling:	How I'm feeling:	How I'm feeling:	How I'm feeling:	How I'm feeling:	How I'm feeling:
Notes:	Notes:	Notes:	Notes:	Notes:	Notes:
Time:	Time:	Time:	Time:	Time:	Time:
Hunger level before:	Hunger level before:	Hunger level before:	Hunger level before:	Hunger level before:	Hunger level before:
Fullness level after:	Fullness level after:	Fullness level after:	Fullness level after:	Fullness level after:	Fullness level after:
Do I feel satisfied?	Do I feel satisfied?	Do I feel satisfied?	Do I feel satisfied?	Do I feel satisfied?	Do I feel satisfied?

JOURNALING TEMPLATE

Use the following questions for times where you are struggling to get into your feelings and need a little prompt. It might also be helpful if your mind is racing before bed and you need to do a 'brain dump'. Or make it a regular practice.

* How am I feeling today?

* What has been going well for me lately?

* What do I need more help/support with?

* What has been weighing on my mind today?

* What do I need to remind myself of in this moment?

* Is there anything I need to do for self-care today?

* What has brought me joy/pleasure today?

* What am I grateful for today?

RESOURCES

For more on the work of the London Centre For Intuitive Eating,
see **@intuitiveeatingldn**, and for more on my work, see
@laurathomasphd and @bub.appetit

Body liberation

@antidietriotclub
@arti.speaks
@benourishpdx
@bodyconfidentmums
@bodyimage_therapist
@bodyposipanda
@bodypositivememes
@comfyfattravels
@curvynyome
@danasuchow
@fit.flexible.fluid
@glitterandlazers
@iamdaniadrianna
@jessicawilson.msrd
@nadia.craddock
@nic.mcdermid
@nicolahaggett
@scarrednotscared
@scotteeisfat
@shooglet
@sofiehagendk

@sonyareneetaylor
@stephanieyeboah
@the_feeding_of_the_fox
@themilitantbaker
@virgietovar
@yourfatfriend

**Intuitive eating and anti-diet
professionals**

@aaronfloresrdn
@alissarumseyrd
@bodypositive_dietitian
@chr1styharrison
@dietitiananna
@elyseresch
@evelyntribole
@fatnutritionist
@foodandfearless
@foodpeacedietitian
@hgoodrichrd
@jennifer_rollin
@lizakhins

@madeonagenerousplan
@marcird
@nourishandeat
@paigesmathersrd
@rebrandedlife
@thedietboycott
@thefuckitdiet
@themindfuldietitian
@thenutritiontea
@vinccird
@wellwitholi
@your.latina.nutritionist
@yourhappyhealthrd

Fitness professionals
@amandalacount
@decolonizingfitness
@janelleyoga
@kanoagreene
@meg.boggs
@missfitsworkout
@mynameisjessamyn
@tallyrye
@thephitcoach
@theunderbellyyoga
@yamalo17

Books on body liberation

Baker, Jes, *Landwhale: On Turning Insults Into Nicknames, Why Body Image Is Hard, and How Diets Can Kiss My Ass* (Seal Press, 2018)

Baker, Jes, *Things No One Will Tell Fat Girls* (Seal Press, 2015)

Cash, Thomas, *The Body Image Workbook: An Eight-Step Program for Learning to Like Your Looks* (2nd Revised Edition: New Harbinger, 2008)

Cooper, Charlotte, *Fat Activism: A Radical Social Movement* (HammerOn Press, 2016)

Crabbe, Megan Jayne, *Body Positive Power: How to stop dieting, make peace with your body and live* (Vermilion, 2017)

Elman, Michelle, *Am I Ugly?* (Anima, 2018)

Hagen, Sofie, *Happy Fat: Taking Up Space in a World That Wants to Shrink You* (Fourth Estate, 2019)

Harding, Kate and Marianne Kirby, *Lessons From the Fat-O-Sphere: Quit Dieting and Declare a Truce with Your Body* (Tarcherperigee, 2009)

MacLean, Roz, *The Body Book* (Promontory Press Inc., 2017)

Miller, Kelsey, *Big Girl: How I Gave Up Dieting and Got a Life* (Grand Central Publishing, 2016)

Sobczak, Connie, *Embody: Learning to Love Your Unique Body (and quiet that critical voice!)* (Gurze Books, 2014)

Taylor, Sonya Renee, *The Body is Not an Apology: The Power of Radical Self-Love* (Berrett-Koehler Publishers, 2018)

Tovar, Virgie, *You Have the Right to Remain Fat* (Melville House UK, 2018)

Wann, Marilyn, *Fat! So?: Because You Don't Have to Apologize for Your Size* (Ten Speed Press, 1998)

West, Lindsey, *Shrill: Notes from a Loud Woman* (Quercus, 2017)

Wolf, Naomi, *The Beauty Myth: How Images of Beauty Are Used Against Women* (Vintage: 1991)

Yeboah, Stephanie, *Fattily Ever After: A Fat, Black Girl's Guide to Living Life Unapologetically* (Hardie Grant, 2020)

Books on health/non-diet nutrition/movement

Bacon, Lindo, and Lucy Aphramor, *Body Respect: What Conventional Health Books Get Wrong, Leave Out, and Just Plain Fail to Understand about Weight* (BenBella Books, 2014)

Bacon, Lindo, *Health At Every Size: The Surprising Truth About Your Weight* (BenBella Books, 2010)

Dooner, Cardine, *The F*ck It Diet: Eating Should Be Easy* (HQ, 2019)

Harrison, Christy, *Anti Diet: Reclaim Your Time, Money, Well-Being and Happiness Through Intuitive Eating* (Little, Brown, 2020)

Levinovitz, Alan, *The Gluten Lie: And Other Myths About What You Eat* (Regan Arts, 2015)

Saunt, Rosie and West, Helen, *Is Butter a Carb? Unpicking Fact from Fiction in the World of Nutrition* (Piatkus, 2019)

Stanley, Jessamyn, *Every Body Yoga* (Workman Publishing, 2017)

Tandoh, Ruby, *Eat Up: Appetite and Eating What You Want* (Serpent's Tail, 2018)

Thomas, Laura, *Just Eat It: How Intuitive Eating Can Help You Get Your Shit Together Around Food* (Bluebird, 2019)

Tribole, Evelyn, and Elyse Resch, *Intuitive Eating: A Revolutionary Program that Works* (Revised Edition: Griffin, 2012)

Tribole, Evelyn, and Elyse Resch, *The Intuitive Eating Workbook: Ten Principles for Nourishing a Healthy Relationship with Food* (New Harbinger, 2017)

Turner, Pixie, *The Wellness Rebel* (Anima, 2018)

Warner, Anthony, *The Angry Chef: Bad Science and the Truth About Healthy Eating* (Oneworld Publications, 2018)

Non-diet/intuitive eating-focused podcasts

Podcasts are an awesome way to feel supported on your intuitive eating journey – download liberally. Don't Salt My Game – this is my podcast, come join us!

Appearance Matters – Nadia Craddock and Jade Parrell

Body Kindness – Rebecca Scritchfield

Body Love Podcast – Jessi Haggerty

The Body Protest – Nadia Craddock and Honey Ross

The Eating Disorder Recovery podcast – Janean Anderson

Eating Words – Sarah Dempster

Food Psych – Christy Harrison

The Full Bloom podcast – Zoë Bisbing and Leslie Bloch

Love, Food – Julie Diffy Dillon

Made of Human – Sofie Hagen

The Mindful Dietitian – Fiona Sutherland

My Black Body – Jessica Wilson and Rawiyah Tariq

Nutrition Matters – Paige Smathers

She's All Fat Pod – April Quioh and Sophia Carter Kahn

Train Happy – Tally Rye

ENDNOTES

INTRODUCTION

1   Tribole E, MS. Definition of Intuitive Eating | Intuitive Eating [Internet]. 2019 [cited 14 May 2020]. Available from: https://www.intuitiveeating.org/definition-of-intuitive-eating/

2   Tribole E, Resch E. *Intuitive Eating*. 3rd ed. St Martin's Griffin; 2012. 320 p.

3   Ledoux T, Daundasekara SS, Beasley A, Robinson J, Sampson M. The association between pre-conception intuitive eating and gestational weight gain. *Eat Weight Disord* – Stud Anorexia, Bulim Obes [Internet]. 3 Mar 2020 [cited 9 Mar 2020]. Available from: http://link.springer.com/10.1007/s40519-020-00878-8

4   Plante AS, Savard C, Lemieux S, Carbonneau É, Robitaille J, Provencher V, et al. Trimester-Specific Intuitive Eating in Association With Gestational Weight Gain and Diet Quality. *J Nutr Educ Behav* [Internet]. 1 Jun 2019 [cited 9 Mar 2020]; 51(6):677–83. Available from: https://linkinghub.elsevier.com/retrieve/pii/S1499404619300259

5   Ciampolini M, Lovell-Smith D, Bianchi R, de Pont B, Sifone M, van Weeren M, et al. Sustained self-regulation of energy intake: initial hunger improves insulin sensitivity. *J Nutr Metab* [Internet]. 22 Jun 2010 [cited 13 Aug 2017] Available from: http://www.ncbi.nlm.nih.gov/pubmed/20721291

6   Schaefer JT, Magnuson AB. A review of interventions that promote eating by internal cues. *J Acad Nutr Diet* [Internet]. 1 May 2014 [cited 17 Apr 2018]; 114(5):734–60. Available from: http://www.ncbi.nlm.nih.gov/pubmed/24631111

7   Soares FLP, Ramos MH, Gramelisch M, de Paula Pego Silva R, da Silva Batista J, Cattafesta M, et al. Intuitive eating is associated with glycemic control in type 2 diabetes. *Eat Weight Disord*. 30 Mar 2020; 1–10.

8   Wheeler BJ, Lawrence J, Chae M, Paterson H, Gray AR, Healey D, et al. Intuitive eating is associated with glycaemic control in adolescents with type I diabetes mellitus. *Appetite* [Internet]. 1 Jan 2016 [cited 8 Apr 2019]; 96:160–5. Available from: http://www.ncbi.nlm.nih.gov/pubmed/26403933

9   Van Dyke N, Drinkwater EJ. Review Article Relationships between intuitive eating and health indicators: literature review. *Public Health Nutr* [Internet]. 21 Aug 2014 [cited 15 Jan 2018]; 17(08):1757–66. Available from: http://www.journals.cambridge.org/abstract_S1368980013002139

10 Tribole E, MS. *Intuitive Eating: Research Update* [Internet]. 2017 [cited 25 Sep 2017]. Available from: https://www.intuitiveeating.org/wp-content/uploads/Intuitive-Eating-Studies-9-18-18.pdf

11   Mensinger JL, Calogero RM, Stranges S, Tylka TL. A weight-neutral versus weight-loss approach for health promotion in women with high BMI: A randomized-controlled trial. *Appetite* [Internet]. Oct 2016 [cited 8 Feb 2019]; 105:364–74. Available from: https://linkinghub.elsevier.com/retrieve/pii/S0195666316302343

12   Carbonneau E, Bégin C, Lemieux S, Mongeau L, Paquette M-C, Turcotte M, et al. A Health at Every Size intervention improves intuitive eating and diet quality in Canadian women. *Clin Nutr* [Internet]. 1 Jun 2017 [cited 19 Apr 2018]; 36(3):747–54. Available from: http://www.ncbi.nlm.nih.gov/pubmed/27378611

13   Tylka TL, Kroon Van Diest AM. The Intuitive Eating Scale–2: Item refinement and psychometric evaluation with college women and men. *J Couns Psychol* [Internet]. 2013 [cited 18 Jul 2017]; 60(1):137–53. Available from: http://doi.apa.org/getdoi.cfm?doi=10.1037/a0030893

14   Humphrey L, Clifford D, Morris MN. Health at Every Size College Course Reduces Dieting Behaviors and Improves Intuitive Eating, Body Esteem, and Anti-Fat Attitudes. *J Nutr Educ Behav*. 2015;47(4).

15   Clifford D, Ozier A, Bundros J, Moore J, Kreiser A, Morris MN. Impact of Non-Diet Approaches on Attitudes, Behaviors, and Health Outcomes: A Systematic Review. *J Nutr Educ Behav* [Internet]. Mar 2015 [cited 20 Nov 2017]; 47(2):143-155.e1. Available from: http://www.ncbi.nlm.nih.gov/pubmed/25754299

16   Hazzard VM, Telke SE, Simone M, Anderson LM, Larson NI, Neumark-Sztainer D. Intuitive eating longitudinally predicts better psychological health and lower use of disordered eating behaviors: findings from EAT 2010–2018. *Eat Weight Disord*. 2020

17   Wilson RE, Marshall RD, Murakami JM, Latner JD. Brief non-dieting intervention increases intuitive eating and reduces dieting intention, body image dissatisfaction, and anti-fat attitudes: A randomized controlled trial. *Appetite*. 1 May 2020;148.

18   Tylka TL, Kroon Van Diest AM. ibid

19   McEnteggart C. A Brief Tutorial on Acceptance and Commitment Therapy as Seen Through the Lens of Derived Stimulus Relations. Vol. 41, *Perspectives on Behavior Science*. Springer International Publishing; 2018. p. 215–27.

CHAPTER 1

1   Harris R. Dropping Anchor: A Script [Internet]. *Act Mindfully*. 2017 [cited 14 May 2020]. Available from: www.ImLearningACT.com

2   Harris R. *Act Made Simple: An Easy-to-Read Primer on Acceptance and Commitment Therapy*. 2nd ed. New Harbinger; 2019. 304 p.

3   McKeever, R. 'Sushi Train Metaphor'. actcursus.nl/wp-content/uploads/2017/04/Sushi-Train-metaphor-Reyelle-McKeever.pdf

4   Harris, R. *The Happiness Trap: Stop Struggling, Start Living*. Robinson Publishing; 2008.

CHAPTER 2

1   Perello M, Sakata I, Birnbaum S, Chuang J-C, Osborne-Lawrence S, Rovinsky SA, et al. Ghrelin increases the rewarding value of high-fat diet in an orexin-dependent manner. *Biol Psychiatry* [Internet]. 1 May 2010 [cited 22 Dec 2017]; 67(9):880–6. Available from: http://www.ncbi.nlm.nih.gov/pubmed/20034618

2   Sobrino Crespo C, Perianes Cachero A, Puebla Jiménez L, Barrios V, Arilla Ferreiro E. Peptides and Food Intake. *Front Endocrinol* (Lausanne) [Internet]. 24 Apr 2014 [cited 4 Jan 2018]; 5:58. Available from: http://journal.frontiersin.org/article/10.3389/fendo.2014.00058/abstract

3   Cummings DE, Weigle DS, Frayo RS, Breen PA, Ma MK, Dellinger EP, et al. Plasma Ghrelin Levels after Diet-Induced Weight Loss or Gastric Bypass Surgery. *N Engl J Med* [Internet]. 23 May 2002 [cited 15 Jun 2018]; 346(21):1623–30. Available from: http://www.nejm.org/doi/abs/10.1056/NEJMoa012908

4   Coutinho SR, Rehfeld JF, Holst JJ, Kulseng B, Martins C. Impact of weight loss achieved through a multidisciplinary intervention on appetite in patients with severe obesity. *Am J Physiol Metab* [Internet]. 23 Jan 2018 [cited 28 May 2018];ajpendo.00322.2017. Available from: http://www.ncbi.nlm.nih.gov/pubmed/29360396

5   Hall KD, Kahan S. Maintenance of Lost Weight and Long-Term Management of Obesity. *Med Clin North Am* [Internet]. Jan 2018 [cited 11 Apr 2019]; 102(1):183–97. Available from: http://www.ncbi.nlm.nih.gov/pubmed/29156185

6   Dirks AJ, Leeuwenburgh C. Caloric restriction in humans: Potential pitfalls and health concerns. *Mech Ageing Dev* [Internet]. Jan 2006 [cited 14 May 2020]; 127(1):1–7. Available from: https://linkinghub.elsevier.com/retrieve/pii/S0047637405002186

7   Stice E, Ng J, Shaw H. Risk factors and prodromal eating pathology. *J Child Psychol Psychiatry* [Internet]. Apr 2010 [cited 5 Apr 2019]; 51(4):518–25. Available from: http://doi.wiley.com/10.1111/j.1469-7610.2010.02212.x

8   Body Confidence Campaign Progress Report 2015 [Internet]. London; Mar 2015 [cited 14 May 2020]. Available from: https://assets.publishing.service.gov.uk/government/uploads/system/uploads/attachment_data/file/417186/Body_confidence_progress_report_2015.pdf

9   Goldstone AP, Prechtl CG, Scholtz S, Miras AD, Chhina N, Durighel G, et al. Ghrelin mimics fasting to enhance human hedonic, orbitofrontal cortex, and hippocampal responses to food. *Am J Clin Nutr*. 1 Jun 2014 ;99(6):1319–30.

10   Fildes A, Charlton J, Rudisill C, Littlejohns P, Prevost AT, Gulliford MC. Probability of an Obese Person Attaining Normal Body Weight: Cohort Study Using Electronic Health Records. *Am J Public Health* [Internet]. Sep 2015 [cited 14 Jan 2019]; 105(9):e54-9. Available from: http://www.ncbi.nlm.nih.gov/pubmed/26180980

11   Truby H, Baic S, deLooy A, Fox KR, Livingstone MBE, Logan CM, et al. Randomised controlled trial of four commercial weight loss programmes in the UK: initial findings from the BBC 'diet trials'. *BMJ* [Internet]. 3 Jun 2006 [cited 2 Oct 2018]; 332(7553):1309–14. Available from: http://www.bmj.com/lookup/doi/10.1136/bmj.38833.411204.80

12   Anderson JW, Konz EC, Frederich RC, Wood CL. Long-term weight-loss maintenance: a meta-analysis of US studies. *Am J Clin Nutr* [Internet]. Nov 2001 [cited 20 Nov 2017]; 74(5):579–84. Available from: http://www.ncbi.nlm.nih.gov/pubmed/11684524

13   Global Weight Management Market Report 2019: Industry Trends, Share, Size, Growth, Opportunity and Forecasts, 2011-2018 & 2019-2024 [Internet]. [cited 14 May 2020]. Available from: https://www.prnewswire.com/news-releases/global-weight-management-market-report-2019-industry-trends-share-size-growth-opportunity-and-forecasts-2011-2018--2019-2024-300948334.html

14   Mental Health Foundation. (2019). *Body Image: How we think and feel about our bodies*. London: Mental Health Foundation.

15   Slater A, Varsani N, Diedrichs PC. #fitspo or #loveyourself? The impact of fitspiration and self-compassion Instagram images on women's body image, self-compassion, and mood. *Body Image* [Internet]. 1 Sep 2017 [cited 9 Feb 2018]; 22:87–96. Available from: https://www.sciencedirect.com/science/article/pii/S1740144516305265?via%3Dihub

16   Turner PG, Lefevre CE. Instagram use is linked to increased symptoms of orthorexia nervosa. *Eat Weight Disord – Stud Anorexia, Bulim Obes* [Internet]. 1 Jun 2017 [cited 18 Jul 2017]; 22(2):277–84. Available from: http://www.ncbi.nlm.nih.gov/pubmed/28251592

17   Slater A, Varsani N, Diedrichs PC. ibid

18   Fatt SJ, Fardouly J, Rapee RM. #malefitspo: Links between viewing fitspiration posts, muscular-ideal internalisation, appearance comparisons, body satisfaction, and exercise motivation in men. *New Media Soc* [Internet]. 1 Jun 2019 [cited 14 May 2020]; 21(6):1311–25. Available from: http://journals.sagepub.com/doi/10.1177/1461444818821064

19   Comiskey, A., Parent, M. C., & Tebbe, E. A. (2020). An inhospitable world: Exploring a model of objectification theory with trans women. *Psychology of Women Quarterly*, 44(1), 105-116.

20   Strübel, J., Sabik, N., & Tylka, T. (2020). Body image and depressive symptoms among transgender and cisgender adults: Examining a Model Integrating the Tripartite Influence Model and Objectification Theory. *Body Image*, 35, 53-62.

21   Brewster, M. E., Sandil, R., DeBlaere, C., Breslow, A., & Eklund, A. (2017). "Do you even lift, bro?" Objectification, minority stress, and body image concerns for sexual minority men. *Psychology of Men & Masculinity*, 18(2), 87.

22   Cohen, R., Newton-John, T., & Slater, A. (2018). 'Selfie'-objectification: The role of selfies in self-objectification and disordered eating in young women. *Computers in Human Behavior*, 79, 68-74.

23   Fardouly, J., Willburger, B. K., & Vartanian, L. R. (2018). Instagram use and young women's body image concerns and self-objectification: Testing mediational pathways. *New Media & Society*, 20(4), 1380-1395.

24   Levinson CA, Fewell L, Brosof LC. My Fitness Pal calorie tracker usage in the eating disorders. *Eat Behav* [Internet]. Dec 2017 [cited 20 Feb 2019]; 27:14–6. Available from: https://linkinghub.elsevier.com/retrieve/pii/S1471015317301484

25 Rentko E. Calorie counting application feedback; potential impact on the teenage female psyche. *J Student Sci Technol* [Internet]. 1 Apr 2015 [cited 11 Mar 2020]; 8(1). Available from: http://journal.fsst.ca/index.php/jsst/article/view/47

26 Mahdawi A. The unhealthy side of wearable fitness devices, Opinion [Internet]. *Guardian*. 2014 [cited 11 Mar 2020]. Available from: https://www.theguardian.com/commentisfree/2014/jan/03/unhealthy-wearable-fitness-devices-calories-eating-disorders-nike-fuelband

27 Simpson CC, Mazzeo SE. Calorie counting and fitness tracking technology: Associations with eating disorder symptomatology. *Eat Behav* [Internet]. Aug 2017 [cited 11 Mar 2020]; 26:89–92. Available from: https://linkinghub.elsevier.com/retrieve/pii/S1471015316303646

CHAPTER 3

1 Richards PS, Crowton S, Berrett ME, Smith MH, Passmore K. Can patients with eating disorders learn to eat intuitively? A 2-year pilot study. *Eat Disord* [Internet]. 15 Mar 2017 [cited 27 Aug 2017]; 25(2):99–113. Available from: https://www.tandfonline.com/doi/full/10.1080/10640266.2017.1279907

2 Garfinkel SN, Seth AK, Barrett AB, Suzuki K, Critchley HD. Knowing your own heart: Distinguishing interoceptive accuracy from interoceptive awareness. *Biol Psychol* [Internet]. 1 Jan 2015 [cited 16 Feb 2018]; 104:65–74. Available from: https://www.sciencedirect.com/science/article/pii/S0301051114002294

3 Herbert BM, Blechert J, Hautzinger M, Matthias E, Herbert C. Intuitive eating is associated with interoceptive sensitivity. Effects on body mass index. *Appetite* [Internet]. Nov 2013 [cited 8 Apr 2019]; 70:22–30. Available from: http://www.ncbi.nlm.nih.gov/pubmed/23811348

4 Tribole E. Intuitive Eating in the Treatment of Eating Disorders: The Journey of Attunement. *Perspect – A Prof J Renfrew Cent Found* [Internet]. 2010 [cited 14 May 2020];Winter. Available from: https://www.evelyntribole.com/wp-content/uploads/Tribole.IntuitiveEating.Eating-Disorders.2010.pdf

CHAPTER 4

1 Brownell KD, Napollitano A. Distorting reality for children: body size proportions of Barbie and Ken dolls. *Int J Eat Disord* [Internet]. 1995 [cited 2020 Jul 18];18(3). Available from: https://pubmed.ncbi.nlm.nih.gov/8556027/

2 Harriger JA, Schaefer LM, Kevin Thompson J, Cao L. You can buy a child a curvy Barbie doll, but you can't make her like it: Young girls' beliefs about Barbie dolls with diverse shapes and sizes. *Body Image* [Internet]. 2019 Sep 1 [cited 2020 Jul 18];30:107–13. Available from: https://pubmed.ncbi.nlm.nih.gov/31238275

3 Piran, Niva. *Journeys of Embodiment at the Intersection of Body and Culture: The Developmental Theory of Embodiment.* Academic Press; 2017

CHAPTER 5

1 Cook-Cottone CP, Guyker WM. The Development and Validation of the Mindful Self-Care Scale (MSCS): an Assessment of Practices that Support Positive Embodiment. *Mindfulness* (N Y) [Internet]. 3 Feb 2018 [cited 20 Feb 2018]; 9(1):161–75. Available from: http://link.springer.com/10.1007/s12671-017-0759-1

2   Nummenmaa L, Hari R, Hietanen JK, Glerean E. Maps of subjective feelings. *Proc Natl Acad Sci U S A.* 11 Sep 2018; 115(37):9198–203.

3   Neff K, Germer C. *Oxford Handbook of Compassion Science* [Internet]. Doty J, editor. Oxford University Press; 2017 [cited 13 Feb 2018]. Available from: http://self-compassion.org/wp-content/uploads/2017/09/Neff.Germer.2017.pdf

4   Albertson ER, Neff KD, Dill-Shackleford KE. *Self-Compassion and Body Dissatisfaction in Women: A Randomized Controlled Trial of a Brief Meditation Intervention.* [cited 13 Feb 2018]; Available from: http://self-compassion.org/wp-content/uploads/publications/AlbertsonBodyImage.pdf

CHAPTER 6

1   Epstein LH, Robinson JL, Temple JL, Roemmich JN, Marusewski A, Nadbrzuch R. Sensitization and habituation of motivated behavior in overweight and non-overweight children. *Learn Motiv* [Internet]. Aug 2008 [cited 22 Mar 2018]; 39(3):243–55. Available from: http://www.ncbi.nlm.nih.gov/pubmed/19649135

2   Myers Ernst M, Epstein LH. Habituation of responding for food in humans. *Appetite* [Internet]. 1 Jun 2002 [cited 22 Mar 2018]; 38(3):224–34. Available from: https://www.sciencedirect.com/science/article/pii/S0195666301904842?via%3Dihub

3   Epstein LH, Fletcher KD, O'Neill J, Roemmich JN, Raynor H, Bouton ME. Food characteristics, long-term habituation and energy intake. Laboratory and field studies. *Appetite* [Internet]. 1 Jan 2013 [cited 13 Feb 2018]; 60:40–50. Available from: https://www.sciencedirect.com/science/article/pii/S0195666312004102

4   Kuznetsova D. *Healthy Places: Councils leading on public health* [Internet]. 2012 [cited 13 Aug 2019]. Available from: http://www.nlgn.org.uk/public/2012/healthy-places-councils-leading-on-public-health/

CHAPTER 8

1   Kabat-Zinn, J., *Full Catastrophe Living* (Piatkus, 2013), pp 15-16

CHAPTER 10

1   Department of Health. Start Active, Stay Active: A report on physical activity from the four home countries' *Chief Medical Officer.* 2011; 62. Available from: https://www.gov.uk/government/uploads/system/uploads/attachment_data/file/216370/dh_128210.pdf

2   NICE. Managing overweight and obesity in adults – lifestyle weight management services. *Public Heal Guid.* 2014; (May):1–79.

3   Saguy AC, Gruys K. Morality and Health: News Media Constructions of Overweight and Eating Disorders. *Soc Probl.* 2010; 57(2):231–50.

4   Hagberg LA, Lindahl B, Nyberg L, Hellénius ML. Importance of enjoyment when promoting physical exercise. *Scand J Med Sci Sport.* 2009; 19(5):740–7.

5   Wankel LM. The importance of enjoyment to adherence and psychological benefits from physical activity. *Int J Sport Psychol.* 1993; Vol 24(2):151–169.

6   Phoenix C, Orr N. Pleasure: A forgotten dimension of physical activity in older age. *Soc Sci Med.* 2014; 115:94–102.

ACKNOWLEDGEMENTS

I want to start out by thanking my clients; you have been my biggest and most important teachers. It's an enormous privilege to learn from you and I will never take for granted how you've entrusted me to support you as you heal your relationship with food. To witness your strength, determination and resilience is inspiring and hands down the best part of my job.

To my team at LCIE; thank you for holding down the fort while I had my *baby* baby and my *book* baby. I'm so proud of you and what we've built together and am so excited for what's next. Love our little gang of nutrition misfits. An extra shoutout to Eliza; I'm pretty sure that copyeditor and babysitter are not in your job description, but I appreciate you stepping up and couldn't have done any of this without your support.

To all of my teachers, mentors, colleagues and other folks who I have had the opportunity to learn from, whether through books, podcasts, social media, conversation or formal training; I am so grateful you have shared your wisdom. A special mention to Fiona Sutherland, Evelyn Tribole, Elyse Resch, Marci Evans, Deb Burgard, Charlotte Cooper, Lindo Bacon, Lucy Aphramor, Christy Harrison, Jessica Wilson, Ragen Chastain, Virgie Tovar, Sonya Renee Taylor, Your Fat Friend, Helen West, Sarah Dempster, Sabrina Springs and many, many more who have dedicated their life's work to building a fairer and more just approach to healthcare. And to the brilliant folks who have contributed to this book; Nikki Haggett, Devinia Noel, Imogen Fox, Scottee, Nadia Craddock, Eliza Khinsoe, Branavie

Ranjithakumaran, Artika Gunathasan, Sofie Hagen, Jess Campbell, Tally Rye, Jake Gifford and Paige Smathers – thank you for lending your voice to this book; your insights and perspectives are incredibly valuable.

To everyone who read *Just Eat It* and has listened to Don't Salt My Game: this book would not have been possible without your incredible support. I am honoured to be a part of your intuitive eating adventure!

A massive thanks to the Bluebird team for letting me write (another!) book and your unwavering support and enthusiasm for my work. And to my literary agent Richard Pike for always having my back.

To my boys; Dave and Avery (Team *Davery!*) – I love you more with each passing day.